Joining the Thin Club

Tips for
Toning Your Mind
After You've
Trimmed Your Body

JOINING
the
THIN CLUB

JUDITH LEDERMAN

AND

LARINA KASE, PSY.D.

Three Rivers Press / New York

Three Rivers Press and the Tugboat design are registered
trademarks of Random House, Inc.

Before photo, page 291: Courtesy of the author
After photo, page 291: LJ Studios; Hair/Makeup, Static Salon

Library of Congress Cataloging-in-Publication Data
Lederman, Judith.
Joining the thin club: tips for toning your mind after you've
trimmed your body / Judith Lederman and Larina Kase.
Includes bibliographical references and index.
1. Weight loss—Psychological aspects—Popular works.
2. Mind and body—Popular works.   I. Kase, Larina.
II. Title.
RM222.2.L39 2007
613.2'5—dc22
2006032557

ISBN 978-0-307-34146-4

Printed in the United States of America

Design by Karen Minster

10 9 8 7 6 5 4 3 2 1

First Edition

To second chances . . .

CONTENTS

JOINING THE THIN CLUB

I SAT AT THE COMMITTEE MEETING AND HEARD THE whispers, again. I'm used to the whispers. "No! *That's* Judy Lederman?? She looks totally different!"

And it's true. I do. I had lost eighty pounds at the time. Eighty pounds makes, quite literally, a mammoth difference in your appearance. It also makes a difference in the way you are perceived by others, but most important, it makes a difference in your mindset. And it isn't always easy to negotiate the feelings that flare up when you are dealing with the psychological ramifications of your weight loss.

There are a few experiences that a former fat person will never forget. Like the time my skinny friend Vicky and I were on a not-too-crowded Metro-North train into the city. It was winter and atop my 225-pound girth, I wore a down-stuffed coat to keep me cozy and warm. We hustled to find a seat before the train filled up, and we came upon a bench seat made for three. A fit executive sat by the window, newspaper spread out, as he leisurely sipped his morning coffee. As I moved into the center seat—next to him—he looked up, surveyed me disdainfully, and sneered, "You've *got* to be kidding!"

I was about to unleash a stream of invectives—after all, I had every right to sit in any vacant seat on the train that I wanted—when skinny Vicky, mortified, pulled me away to another seat, where we endured the ride hunched next to the smelly toilet.

It didn't take long for me to stop sitting in public places. I was afraid of breaking the folding chairs. And forget the buffet table. There was no way I was going to let anyone see Fat Ole Me scarfing down stuffed cabbage or, worse, pastries at a party.

What a difference a few years and a few pounds can make. Now when I go on the train I still feel eyes on me as I choose a seat, although the reactions I'm likely to get now are not mean at all. They are friendly gazes inviting me to sit down. Sometimes after I sit, the person alongside me strikes up a friendly conversation. I've been accepted into The Thin Club.

And while in some ways it is infinitely more comfortable to get these reactions, it is all so new to me. And there is a new edge. In my mind, when I scrutinize myself in the mirror, I'm still—and will likely *always* be—the fat lady I once was. And while I'm thrilled to fit into a size 8 and I know I've worked hard to get there, there's a part of me that is a little insulted that people were—and still are—so influenced by my outer appearance. "What, *now* you like me?" I think to myself. "I'm still the same person I was, aren't I? Why did you not want to take the time to get to know me when I was heavy?"

And here's the real kicker. Now when I see an overweight person—sometimes in spite of all I've been through or maybe because of it—I find myself slipping into a new frame of mind: a "Thin Club" mentality. There's a part of me that judges overweight people and wonders why they choose to bury themselves in Oreos instead of hitting the treadmill. And even though I catch myself in horror—after all, it hasn't been that long since I've had a decadently intimate relationship with a Valrhona Fudge Mousse Pecan Torte drizzled with crème fraîche—there's a smugness about being part of my new club, even though I don't always believe that I'm a member.

Although I now belong, and am newly single, there's another part of me that still doesn't know how to handle compliments, sexual comments, and appraising looks. I sometimes find it more comfortable to hide behind sunglasses and bulky jackets than sport body-hugging clothes.

For most of my life I was fat, and most days I battled the attitudes of others as well as my own shaky self-image. Would you believe that at 225 pounds I had *fat-blindness,* in that I looked in the mirror as a fat person and didn't see someone all that fat. Denial is a cushion that this derriere found way too comfortable! And I was in denial—big time! Only in the glaring lights of the large-size women's department dressing rooms, when I realized that even a size 20 was crimping my ever-burgeoning waist, and eventually on the cold steel table of an operating room where doctors performed an angiogram to assess the damage I might have done to my poor overfed heart, did I face the fact that I was heavy. But as confusing as fat was, now that I'm thinner things are even more confusing.

Reconciling the inner me with the outer "new" me has been a difficult task and has required a new and improved attitude on my part. While some things have changed for the better, others—like the blissful indulgence of alternating melting bites of a sweet ice cream sundae with salty corn chips—have fallen by the wayside. And while I can't honestly say I miss the gastric complaints or sugar highs, and the inevitable mood crashes and vegetative states, that went along with unfettered feeding, there are times when I miss the basic act of just eating whatever I want without all the intellectualizing, inner proselytizing, umpteen explanations, exercise planning, and guilt that goes along with it.

Since I joined The Thin Club so much has happened. I left an abusive and painful marriage after twenty-two years, leaving people to snipe, "She got thin, sexy, and left her poor husband in the dust!" But becoming thin wasn't the impetus for this change. Becoming strong was the catalyst. As I became stronger in body, mind, and spirit, I was able to face the myriad problems in my marriage; the new, thin me said, "Yes, you *can* make it on your own, scary as that might be. You don't deserve to be punished—you should be honored and cared for!"

Why do so many people who finally lose the weight quickly put it back on? Could it be that their emotional and intellectual "shapes" need as much exercise as their brand-new bodies? And what about those who don't even bother losing the weight? Is it possible that they know in their heart of hearts that even if they take the weight off, the problems that made them heavy to begin with are harder to shed than the pounds?

With weight-loss surgeries becoming a new option, and dramatic and fast weight loss becoming entirely possible, more people than ever are finding themselves members of The Thin Club. And while most of them enjoy their new wardrobes and the admiring looks they get from others, not all of them have enough internal strength to get past the initiation rites.

Is losing weight really all it's cracked up to be? One woman I met who had undergone gastric bypass surgery had nothing nice to say about food anymore, even though she had achieved significant weight loss. She no longer enjoys food the way she did when she was fat. She misses indulging in huge portions of layer cake and even regrets her weight loss. Or maybe she just wasn't ready to join The Thin Club.

An attractive pediatrician who lost a lot of weight by

dieting says that a day doesn't go by when she doesn't scrutinize the mirror, seeking some validation as she tries to assure herself that there really *is* a difference be-tween her former face, wreathed in roundness, and her former size 18 body, and her new delicate, high-cheeked appearance and size 6 persona. "I just don't see what everyone else is talking about," she confides. "I just see the bra bulges and catch myself eating things I shouldn't all the time."

Thinking thin hardly comes naturally to someone who has been overweight for a long time. We're only as good as our last well-planned, low-calorie, low-carb, sugar-free, or point-controlled meal. And that may explain why, accord-ing to the National Institutes of Health, 95 percent of peo-ple who lose large amounts of weight tend to regain it within the first three years of losing it. The number is smaller with patients who have lost weight through surgery, but it is still significant.

Just as our bodies need sculpting when we finally reach a weight near our goal, our minds need molding to accom-modate the new, thin person within. There have been so many new lessons on the way down and into the ranks of The Thin Club. The challenges are numerous, but I face them with strength and excitement—and you can, too.

Know that although statistics show that the vast major-ity of people who lose weight tend to regain it, there are others who have maintained their weight loss by changing their lifestyles and behaviors. By seizing control, you stand a better chance of controlling your body. But of course there are certain things that are dictated to us by our bodies—our genetic makeup, our metabolism, our flexi-bility, and our general health.

I met Dr. Larina Kase, a Philadelphia-based psycholo-gist and success coach specializing in anxiety and weight loss, while we were both appearing on *The Jane Pauley Show*. The show was about the "downside" of weight loss. There can be a downside? you ask. Anyone who has done it will agree—there can be and *is* a downside. Weight-loss problems are vast and old habits die hard. I talked about my problems: about the bittersweet excitement of negotiating store racks and not knowing how to shop, about mourning the years I spent fat, and about learning to adjust my "personal space meter" to not take wide strides to accommodate my perceived (but no longer real) girth. Larina, an expert on the thoughts, behaviors, and feelings associated with weight loss, who at the time was a clinician at the University of Pennsylvania, analyzed me in front of the television audience: "There is a period of time in which the mind has to catch up with the body. It just has trouble accepting its new sleek contours—and while everyone else sees 'thin,' the fat person peers back from the other side of the mirror at someone who has lost weight."

She was right. The studio audience was incredulous to hear that I had trouble accepting my size 6/8 self, and that I still saw my body oozing out of a size 24 when I looked in the mirror. They applauded me, but it was hard to accept the praise. Jane looked at me and said, "I can't believe that, after all the progress you have made, you see only the negative side of your appearance."

The "Are We There Yet?" mentality is one of the biggest problems for many of us who are losing or have lost weight. We just don't recognize where we were and how far we've come. In our quest for the whole enchilada, we don't enjoy the appetizers along the way; instead, we frequently sabotage ourselves and send ourselves back to the starting gate.

When I spoke to Larina after the show, we agreed that if I was having trouble with the post-weight-loss issues, chances are so were others. In fact, Larina had been approached by many clients for weight-loss coaching *after* they'd lost the weight. And with that, the concept for The Thin Club, this book, and our website, www.thethinclub .com, went from idea to reality.

While many books share the "secrets" of diet success, none explores the fear, the mixed emotions, and the uneasiness that are frequently odd side effects of a successful weight loss. After dealing with the emotions that dogged me as I fought my way downscale, I was compelled to talk about them. Initially, my revelations that skinny doesn't always feel successful didn't win me much sympathy. But as I began to talk to other former fat people, I found that I wasn't alone. We all seemed to have a deep, dark secret that we carried around. Many were afraid to talk about it— afraid of the eye rolling and the "yeah, right!" comments they would inspire. As a writer and a public speaker, I realized that I was in a unique position. I could explore my own feelings and help others at the same time. What better way to address and conquer the diet demons?

After interviewing others and dealing with my own feelings, I decided to write about some of the more common fears, gripes, and challenges that are bound to creep up on someone who is losing or has lost weight. I share with you my story and the secrets I have learned on my journey downscale, and Larina provides tips on how to handle the challenges that lurk in the dark recesses of your refrigerator—and at Costco in family-size containers of greasy snacks. Because those challenges, external as they are, are really internal, and in order to live well and at maximum energy and vitality, we need to confront them.

THE THIN CLUB MEMBERSHIP

Losing weight is one of the most difficult things that there is to do. Successful weight loss results from a complex interaction of behavioral, mental, and emotional changes. Whether you lost weight by a combination of eating modifications and exercise or by surgical or other medical interventions, the process is tough. You know this. You've made it to The Thin Club? Or have you?

You may have heard about this book or had it in hand, wondering if it will apply to you. If you've lost a significant amount of weight, then it does apply to you. Let's begin by taking a look at who will succeed in The Thin Club.

We know how to diet—we've done it—and it doesn't matter how we lost the weight. We are success stories, right? The proof is in the sugar-free pudding! What is the "fooditude" of someone who has lost weight?

Have Thin Club members resigned themselves to forever ban sweets and munchies from their lives? What creates cravings and can we honestly keep them out of our lives, once and for all? Has dieting created a "fear of enjoying food"? Will we ever be able to eat like a thin person (even though we *are* thin)? Can we ever hope to put a morsel in our mouths without thinking about it? Thin Club members tend to focus on "living to eat" versus "eating to live" and that attitude enables "big fat losers" to stay focused on living as thin persons. What are some of the best-kept secrets of members of The Thin Club?

CHALLENGES INVOLVED
WITH WEIGHT-LOSS SURGERY

A common area of criticism and debate is weight-loss surgery. If you have had this surgery, know someone who has, or are contemplating it, you probably also know about some of the biases that people have. People (maybe even you) often think that surgery is "cheating" or taking the easy way out. Has anyone ever said this to you? Have you ever heard or thought that weight-loss surgery is less impressive than weight loss the "natural" way?

If you've lost weight, chances are good that everyone asks you how you did it. Often, the "wow factor" is not as strong when you say you had surgery as when you say you did the good old-fashioned diet and exercise routine. The reason for this is that most people who try to lose weight through diet and exercise are not successful, either at losing the weight or at keeping it off. When you say you accomplished your weight loss through these means, they are impressed because you've done what they haven't been able to do. But when you say that you lost weight through surgery, people cannot relate as well. They don't understand the difficulties you faced and the challenges you had to overcome.

People have an idealized view of weight-loss surgery: you go in, you lose 100 pounds, and life is great and easy. Well, it isn't so easy. People don't always understand all the preparation you had to do for the surgery and all the changes you endured post-op. They don't know what it's like to only eat a half cup of food at a time; adjust to new emotions, relationships, and body image; and dramatically change your lifestyle in a short period of time.

Tammy St. Clair, a thirty-five-year-old woman who lost over eighty pounds after a lap-band procedure, explains that lap-band patients have to adjust to an entirely new regimen of eating, in terms of not just *what* they eat but also *how* they eat. "Post-lap-band-surgery eating requires focusing on taking tiny bites, chewing slowly, and careful swallowing," she says. "That makes it particularly difficult to do in public places—parties, restaurants."

While she describes similar adjustments to the emotional factors of her weight loss—acknowledgment of her "thin" self, the shock of no longer feeling "invisible," the way she describes herself in her former fat state—her food-related challenges differ slightly from those of people whom lose weight through diet and exercise. Tammy now runs monthly lap-band support groups in a Westchester County, New York, mall food court for others who are in the process of losing weight. She says this support helps her members focus on eating in a public place full of distractions, but it also gives them a climate-controlled environment where they can walk for exercise and share stories of their common challenges.

TIP

Remember, losing weight is the only requirement for membership in The Thin Club. As long as you used a healthy method—such as changing your eating habits, developing a new lifestyle, or exercising—or had weight-loss surgery, you are a bona fide member (read: we don't approve of eating-disorder strategies, such as starving yourself or purging). Own your membership and don't let anyone convince you that you don't deserve it. No matter which strategy you used to lose weight, it was difficult. You've earned your membership. What we care about is that you stay in The Thin Club!

Because of the struggles that people go through with weight-loss surgery, Larina and a colleague who lost half her body weight with bariatric surgery developed an entire coaching program to work through the process of weight-loss surgery. We know that it is a difficult process to lose weight *no matter how you do it!*

This book contains tips from the trenches—from women and men who have joined The Thin Club, however they happened to attain membership—and for those who plan on staying a member for some time.

WHO IS MOST LIKELY TO SUCCEED IN THE THIN CLUB?

You are most likely to succeed in The Thin Club when you:

1. Believe that you belong.
2. Work on changing some of your thoughts, feelings, and behaviors to those most likely to keep you in The Thin Club.
3. Look in the mirror and finally see . . . well . . . someone attractive and not *fat!*

DO I DESERVE TO BE A MEMBER OF THE THIN CLUB?

Believing that you belong in The Thin Club is critical to ensuring your membership for life. You may be wondering how much weight you need to have lost or how thin you need to be as a member. Unfortunately many people who would certainly be included in The Thin Club because they have lost a substantial amount of weight don't include themselves because they think they don't deserve it.

In clinical studies, the goal for weight loss at the end of treatment is typically around 10 percent of your initial body weight. For example, if you started off at 180 pounds, a weight-loss goal after several months of your program would be around eighteen pounds. You may think that this is not enough weight to lose to be considered eligible for

The Thin Club. But this thought process is a mistake, and it may be setting you up to gain the weight back. If your weight loss is a "success" by clinical standards, then you need to see it as a personal success as well and use that sense of achievement to motivate you to further lose weight or maintain the weight you've lost.

We are certainly not advocating a Thin Club consisting only of 110-pound women and 160-pound men. Instead, it is meant for those who have successfully lost a significant amount of weight and wish to keep it off or to continue their weight loss. You don't have to be a supermodel. You don't have to be perfect. But you do need to feel good about the weight you've lost. If you undervalue the weight loss you have achieved, you are more likely to abandon your weight-loss or maintenance efforts.

TIP

Believing that you belong is one of the first steps. We will focus on the success, joy, and victories of weight loss throughout this book rather than get caught up in insecurities, fears, and failure. Begin your Thin Club membership by writing a list of all the reasons you deserve to be a member and how you have earned your membership. Once you're convinced you're a bona fide member, you'll start enjoying all the benefits of membership. Read on . . .

THE BENEFITS OF MEMBERSHIP

Everybody knows about the multiple benefits of weight loss. The health benefits, including biological, psychological, and relationship improvements, are vast. Obesity is linked with dozens of health problems, including cardiovascular disease, certain cancers, diabetes, hypertension, osteoarthritis, and other musculoskeletal problems. Weight loss reduces your risks of developing these health problems.

Psychologically, one of the greatest benefits associated with entering The Thin Club is an enhanced quality of life. Studies typically show an improved quality of life following weight loss for those who have lost weight by dieting or surgery. These improvements are likely to be responsible for consequent improvements in mood and anxiety levels.

For example, researchers followed people who had bariatric surgery. Before surgery, their scores on almost all measures of quality of life were lower than people of normal weight. Following surgery, their scores on all scales increased to equivalent to or higher than the averages for those of normal weight.

Other benefits to entering The Thin Club can include improved relationships, enhanced self-esteem, and better mood and energy.

THE COSTS OF MEMBERSHIP

Obviously there are a ton of benefits to being in The Thin Club. That's why you worked so hard to get here. But these benefits don't always happen, or they happen later than you expected, or they are less intense and less life-changing than you expected. People don't talk about the aftermath of weight loss. They don't discuss the difficulty of toning your mind once you've toned your body. They assume that life will be great and problem free after the weight loss. But membership in The Thin Club has fees you need to pay.

Up-front Membership Fees

The biggest upfront fee is the work that you've done to get into the club. You may have limited your eating to 1,400 calories of healthy food per day. You might have become a permanent fixture in your gym. Maybe you cut out carbs and subsisted without your beloved ice cream or bagels for six months. Or you may have undergone months of evaluation, surgical procedures, recovery, and diet modification. Regardless of the method that helped you enter The Thin Club, you surely paid your dues.

Ongoing Membership Dues

Unfortunately your dues are not paid up with the up-front costs. To remain a member, there will be some ongoing costs. After successful weight loss with one of the most effective treatments for obesity, behavioral therapy, most people regain the weight within three years. According to the Institute of Medicine, those who lose 10 percent of their body weight regain two-thirds of the weight lost within one year and almost all of it within five years. These figures are depressing, unless you know what to do to stay in The Thin Club.

TIP

Realize that staying in The Thin Club takes some work. There are up-front fees and ongoing dues, but it is worth it! If you're clear on why you want to keep your weight off and you stay motivated, then staying in the club won't feel like work. You need to expect it to be difficult and challenging at times, but you can remind yourself why it's so important to forge ahead.

Think of the journey as an airplane flight with some turbulence. There are some smooth times, some beautiful views, and some nice people near you. There are also rocky and choppy times, irritating people around you, and times when it feels like the flight is taking forever. But when you reach your destination and get to enjoy being there, you will want to stay there forever.

Many people do not make the mental, behavioral, and relationship changes necessary to keep weight off. They then suffer the emotional turmoil that comes with regaining weight. Research suggests that to ensure long-term weight loss, you must have realistic goals about your weight, address your body-image concerns, and consistently adhere to a healthy diet and exercise plan.

THIN CLUB THINKING

Almost everyone who embarks on a weight-loss treatment has unrealistic expectations for how much weight she or he can lose and how quickly that will happen. Studies show that the mismatch between expectation and actual loss leads to demoralization and lack of adherence to a program. This means that if you have lost weight, but you are dwelling on the fact that it isn't as much weight as you want to lose, you may be in trouble. To maintain your weight loss you will need to overcome specific internalized standards, like the feeling that you need to have the "ideal" body.

Another thought process that is necessary to staying thin is banishing derogatory self-statements. Many overweight men and women get into the habit of negatively critiquing themselves. You may be aware of your tendencies to do this. Or it may be so second nature that you don't even notice. Once a thought pattern is in place, it is very tough to break. If you are in the habit of linking your weight with your self-esteem, you may develop an unhealthy obsession with your weight. If you gain a pound, your self-esteem is at risk to plummet. If these negative habits and self-statements persist, they may sabotage your ability to stay in The Thin Club.

FAT CLUB TEMPTATIONS

One of the major difficulties in remaining a Thin Club member is that many of your actions and behaviors may not have changed. You are likely to be in the same environment as you were in when you were heavier. Or your habits may have changed temporarily, only to revert back under times of stress or when your weight-loss goal is gone.

For instance, many people who have lost weight find themselves still around high-fat foods. These foods are everywhere! You sit down in front of a giant box of sugary, tempting donuts that's on the table in a meeting at work. Your husband brings home a take-out meal of Chinese food. You walk into a movie theater and become overwhelmed with the buttery, salty smell of freshly popped popcorn. It is hard to live a life away from temptations. But these temptations may tempt you right out the door of The Thin Club and into The Fat Club, if you aren't careful.

We aren't suggesting that you not go to the movies because of the smell of popcorn, but we do recommend that you carefully think about your behavioral patterns and consider what can be changed. We will help you to do this.

EXERCISE YOUR MEMBERSHIP

While exercise is not the most efficient way to lose weight (without changing eating habits, exercise alone tends to lead to slow weight loss), many studies have shown that it is crucial for keeping weight off. Those who are active keep their membership activated.

In one study, regular physical activity was reported by 90 percent of those who kept their weight off. In contrast, only 34 percent of those who regained the weight reported regular exercise. The researchers concluded that physical activity is an important maintenance factor for healthy body weight, both for those who have lost weight and for "normal" weight individuals.

Inspired to keep moving? We'll go through what you need to know about exercising your Thin Club membership.

TIP

Continuously tone your mind and body. One of the principles of The Thin Club is that you tone your mind along with your body. Don't worry if you don't know how to do that yet—that's why you're reading the book. We'll help you. For now, commit to the idea of an ongoing process of mind and body toning and read on . . .

Thin Club membership begins the day you make a commitment to lose the weight and it continues long after you have experienced the bittersweet joy of being a "loser." For those still on the road to losing, there are times you'll reach a plateau in your weight loss and feel like giving up. Throughout this book, we reveal the secrets of staying in The Thin Club.

SECRETS TO STAYING A MEMBER

You've lost weight—that's wonderful! Joining the club is one thing. But staying in the club is not so easy. You may have lost and regained weight in the past. If you haven't experienced this yourself, surely you know people who have been trapped in the dreaded yo-yo dieting cycle. Most of us have.

The process of regaining the weight you have lost takes a tremendous toll on you, physically and emotionally. The frustration and even hopelessness that occur when you regain the weight that you worked so hard to lose is intense. In this book, you'll be learning some of the top methods that have helped people to keep weight off.

One of our goals in writing this book is to help you be thin or thinner than you once were—not just temporarily but also for life. As for any club, the goal of The Thin Club is to have members for the long term, not just the short term. You can really begin to adjust to and enjoy the "new you," not the "temporary you." We want to help you end that frustrating process of regaining weight or of living in fear of regaining the weight. To maintain your weight loss, it is important to have realistic goals about your weight, address body-image concerns, and adhere to a plan for healthy diet and exercise.

Joining the Thin Club is not a diet book. You will learn weight-loss secrets—my own journey of how I lost weight as well as the experiences of others—including the thoughts, feelings, emotional revelations, and obstacles that frequently occur on the way "downscale." While there are already an infinite number of "diet books" out there, this is more of an après diet book, meaning it helps people who have already peeled off some pounds to stay on course, adjust to their new bodies, understand why they may have been fat to begin with, maintain their high activity levels, and deal with the new and unsettling reactions they are likely getting from others.

The stressors that cause someone to pack on weight don't just magically disappear when the weight is gone. Learning how to identify those stressors, combat them using means other than food, and deal with the issues that are bound to surface once weight is no longer a factor in your life is one of the tools you will walk away with after reading this book.

We will explain the various stages of weight loss, give tips for adjusting to each stage of the process, and share mental and physical exercises to help your mind catch up with the progress that your body has made. We also report on interviews with people in various stages of dealing with these issues and the views of experts who can shed light on the reasons for these challenges and how to tackle them.

Oprah Winfrey, Kirstie Alley, Carnie Wilson, and many others have fought to become members but not everyone has managed to stay in the club. Learn now how you can attain and, more important, retain membership. Welcome to The Thin Club!

ONE

AGAINST ALL ODDS

How I Made the Journey Downscale

The Question I Get Asked Most:
How Did You Lose the Weight?

HINT: It's *Not* About the Diet!

FOR YEARS I HAD TURNED UP MY NOSE AT THE MERE thought of a diet. I was, without question, the most unmotivated person on the planet. Once in a while, though, life has a strange way of giving you a well-placed kick. Mine came in the form of an angiogram.

The day I sat in a wheelchair, in a bleak foyer outside the operating room suite, I was forced to face the consequences of a lifetime of neglect. I was barefoot and my thin hospital gown was barely covered by a threadbare hospital-issue blanket.

My forty-year-young heart just couldn't be clogged. True, it had been broken once or twice many years before, but clogged arteries? The doctor I hadn't seen in three years had obviously thought I was doomed. I had been getting "arm squeezes"—pressure that started in my left arm and radiated into my chest. I was finding it hard to walk, go up steps, and exert myself at all. One day the pressure got extreme and I went to the doctor. He gave me an aspirin and checked me into the NYU Emergency Room. He thought I might be having a heart attack.

OK, so I'm a workaholic. I see myself more as a "precision-timed juggler," keeping my three children, my busy public relations business, my radio show, my writing, my then husband, and all the other flora and fauna of a late baby boomer's life somehow in sync—at least most of the time. Time for myself rarely enters the picture. When I do find a moment to rest, I usually remember something I forgot to do, like go to the bathroom. Taking long walks in the woods? That's for narcissists! I could never be so ridiculously indulgent! Exercise class? Another time-waster. Or so I thought then.

Until the angiogram, I always ate on the run, grabbing whatever was easiest—french fries, pizza, pasta, any kind of bagel, cake, or muffin. Salad took way too much time to shop for and even more time to prepare. And it tasted yucky. I watched the scale topping out at 220+ pounds, but I didn't much care because I never even had time to look in the mirror. And when I did, I never saw myself as fat!

But now I was seated on a gurney in the Emergency Room of the hospital, and a cardiologist pulled the privacy drapes around me. "If you let me out of here now, I swear I'll never eat another french fry," I pleaded, not quite sure I could ever make good on that promise. "I'll even give up chocolate."

"Heavens, you will not give up chocolate!" he laughed. "You can still have chocolate—just not a whole lot of it!"

So here I was, awaiting an angiogram and wondering how the outcome would affect my life. And how many Valrhona chocolates were left in my future.

"Don't you have slippers?" The nurse looked at my bare feet.

"I came straight from work." I shrugged.

She found me some paper booties, and I shuffled from the gurney into what looked like an operating room and felt like a meat locker. I began to shake from the cold. She helped me onto an even colder table and barely covered me with the thin blanket. In spite of the blindingly bright lights, I was shivering and my teeth were chattering. Another nurse wrapped a tourniquet around my arm, tying it shut with the snapping of rubber against rubber.

"This will pinch a bit," she warned as she stuck me with an IV needle.

"Dang," she swore as she missed the vein. She maneuvered the needle around, causing shards of pain to course through my arm. I jumped as someone clipped a pulse monitor to my toe and as someone else began lowering the blanket from my groin. A short and chubby nurse leaned over the table nonchalantly.

"I have to shave you," she said, brandishing the razor.

There I was—control fiend, workaholic, and nurturer— prostrate on an uncomfortable table, completely dependent on doctors and nurses who were giving me a free "Brazilian." Dean Koontz and Stephen King combined couldn't come up with a more horrific scenario.

The first nurse had given up on the initial vein she had chosen and was hunting for another, this time in my forearm. "I used to be real good at this," she muttered, as I tried not to squirm. Finally she gave up and asked the doctor to try his hand at it.

"You have one last chance," I warned him. "And then I'm outta here. I'm not a pincushion, you know."

He didn't look too worried. He knew I wouldn't get far. In one swift motion, he threaded the IV into my vein. Pay dirt. I don't know what was in the IV, but I soon stopped shivering. My relief was short-lived, as the chubby nurse poked a syringe into my IV tube and squeezed. An instant, blood-chilling sting suffused my arm.

"Benadryl." She shrugged as I yelped.

"If you say 'I told you so!' we're history," I had said as I glared at my husband. The last thing I wanted to do was give this husband of mine—the one who preferred salad to his own birthday cake—the satisfaction of being right.

He had shrugged helplessly before he was asked to leave the ER. And now, here I lay on the table in the freezing cold cath lab as two doctors, dressed in matching turquoise scrub suits, huddled over my pelvis. She was blonde and blue-eyed. He was tall and slim. They looked like Dr. Barbie and nuclear cardiologist Ken, getting ready for a heart-stopping adventure in my femoral artery.

"This is the only part you'll feel," Dr. Ken promised. Pain spread through my pelvis as he injected me with a local anesthetic.

Then I felt the sickening sensation of blood dripping down my hip and over my inner thigh. The doctors were studying the screens as they threaded the catheter up toward my heart. They talked to each other in hushed tones. I couldn't quite make out what they were saying. I would have liked to know more about the procedure and what they were looking at, but I didn't want to sound the way my kids do when we go on a road trip.

"Hey, Docs, are we there yet?"

I felt like a live cadaver as Barbie and her friend whispered to one another. My feelings of helplessness awakened my worst fears, and my fertile imagination began to work overtime. I imagined their hushed conversation.

"The stupid fool has obviously been eating french fries more than once a week." Dr. Barbie wrinkles her nose in disgust. I'm shaken out of my reverie by the real sound of Dr. Barbie's voice.

"In a few seconds you're going to feel a burning sensation in your chest. That's the dye we're injecting. It will spread to the rest of your body after it goes through your heart."

Burning? Try searing, flaming, incandescent, ablaze— those words more aptly describe the sensation of the dye going through my system. My heart was afire and the rest of me wasn't far behind. The fire spread to my groin and feet and arms. Then my heart started skipping beats. Am I dying? Is this the "big one"? I'm choked with fear and I think of my children. I'm never going to see them again. I'm going to expire here in the cath lab.

"That's going to stop soon," Dr. Barbie assured me. How did she know my heart was doing those things? "How do you know it'll stop?" I asked her.

"We've got it under control," she responded.

Was this a hospital or a medieval torture chamber? What's next, the rack?

I must have accidentally voiced my thoughts aloud because she replied, "Wait, you haven't even seen the recovery room."

"Good news, though," she assured me. "Your heart is just fine. There's no blockage in any of your arteries."

Thank you, God! I was a death-row inmate receiving a presidential pardon. I thought about the saucy Chinese food, eggplant-topped pizza, enormous kosher deli sandwiches, mounds and mounds of Ben & Jerry's Chubby-Hubby ice cream, french fries, french fries, and more french fries I had been desecrating my body with. I didn't deserve a second chance, but somehow I'd gotten one.

I didn't even wince when the nurse pushed more Benadryl through my IV tube.

For me, suffering through the angiogram was like peering through a window into my future. If I continued the way I'd been going, I was bound to end up back in the cath lab someday. Maybe it would take twenty years, or maybe forty, but somehow I knew I'd be back and that next time I may not get to go back to work the next day.

It was at that precise moment that I invented the "I Never Want Another Angiogram (as long as I live) Diet." It's simple and easy to follow. There are no gimmicks, pills, or magic potions. Eat healthy, eat right, and when you're tempted by Junior's Cheesecake, crispy french fries, or mouthwatering Belgian truffles, reread this chapter and visualize the cath lab. Imagine just for one moment the feeling of hot dye burning through your veins. That was me, but it could just as easily have been you. No diet works without a powerful motivator, and I for one am not likely to forget that angiogram anytime soon.

That angiogram started me on a program of self-realization, and the self-realization led to a drastic lifestyle change. I realized that losing weight is not about food at all. The key is changing your attitude—hearing the wake-up call and deciding "enough is enough." I was ready to be thin. No more excuses for gaining weight or staying unhappily static. I took responsibility for my nutrition, my fitness, my overall health, and my life as a whole.

The new me is a lot like my ex-husband. I cut carbs, refuse sugar, embrace exercise, and make very careful choices. It's been ten years since I started the diet, and I've lost over ninety pounds since my angiogram. I've reclaimed my life. No french fry can compare with the joy of an easy zip on a size 8 pair of jeans, especially when I once was a size 22 with an elastic waistband. And I have learned to find pleasure in things other than food. Walks in the woods are *not* frivolous at all, and exercise makes me feel good, healthy, and sexy, so I make time for it each day. I'm worth it!

There was a casualty back in that hospital. Martyr mom, the victimized woman who did everything for everyone but very little for herself, died that day on the angiogram table. The new me is a victim no more.

THE DIET

There are so many different diets and methods of losing weight these days, from surgical procedures to Overeaters Anonymous to the tried-and-true Weight Watchers. It doesn't really matter *how* you lose it. Simply put, calories in should not exceed calories out. That is the hallmark of every good diet. But anyone who has ever had a weight problem knows that this is easier said than done. When presented with bread to nibble on at a restaurant or running past a donut stand after skipping breakfast, most people will find themselves mindlessly munching. Is there really such a thing as mindless munching? There shouldn't be.

And there isn't for me anymore. Sugar is a four-letter word in my household. In purging much of it from my cupboard, my life, and my body, I have succeeded in quelling cravings that used to haunt me, whether the sugar perpetrator was a bag of baby carrots or a Snickers bar. There are some foods that will never be welcome in my body. I accept and embrace that aesthetic fact. It's OK. I no longer miss it.

I don't diet. *Diet* means inherently counting calories, points, measuring foods. Instead, I feed my body what it needs when it needs it. It doesn't *need* or *want* a candy bar or piece of mousse cake. Ever. So I don't bother with empty calories. I have learned that life holds delights far more lasting and enjoyable than the fleeting pleasure of sugar melting on my tongue. And in fact, the "sugar high" is accompanied by energy and mood surges that affect my overall mood, usually in a colossal end "crash."

According to Harold Schulman, a medical doctor and professor at the State University of New York–Stony Brook, the food-mood connection is not a fluke, and balance is the key to maintaining even moods. He explains that we start out life with the perfect food—mother's milk. It has 45 percent carbohydrate, 30 percent protein, and the rest fat. A balanced meal. What happens next is that nature turns to nurture—for example, mother and the media take over. The milk becomes secondary and the basic message of carbohydrate, protein, and fat balance is lost. Taste becomes the driving force.

TIP

Stay balanced. We need carbohydrates. They are our best source of energy, and the brain uses only carbs to function. But balance your carb intake with adequate protein to avoid sugar surges.

WHICH COMES FIRST? THE FOOD OR THE MOOD?

According to Dr. Schulman, the two valuable research areas for food and mood are serotonins and carbohydrates. We know that serotonin is a brain messenger that signals when we are full or satisfied. In the 1990s, there was a drug called fenfluramine, part of a combo fen-phen that was the most powerful and effective pill ever found for losing weight. Millions of people saw their excess weight melt away. The pill diminished their hunger; they felt full sooner, were happier, and gained energy. Unfortunately for some people the increases in serotonin affected the heart and lungs. Fen-phen was promptly taken off the market.

There are two building blocks for making serotonin: protein and carbohydrate. In the protein, there has to be an amino acid called tryptophan. The tryptophan piggy-backs onto the carbohydrate and provides the essential ingredients for making serotonin. Oftentimes at the end of a meal we crave something sweet. According to Dr. Schulman, this could be habit or your body asking for an ingredient like a little carbohydrate to boost the serotonin production. Because our appetite brain center is near the energy and mood centers, food is a natural means for boosting mood, and it is done through the balance of protein and carbs.

This explains why empty calories used to make me sluggish: They sapped my energy. Excess sugar in my system created a high and then a crash that would frequently leave me depressed and exhausted—too exhausted to move around much. The technical term for this condition, according to J. Shah, a physician board-certified in the field of bariatric (weight-loss) medicine, is "food coma" or "sugar crash." There really is a food-mood connection—the drowsiness and lethargy induced by eating too much or eating foods that aren't nutritionally balanced.

Dr. Shah says that "zoned out" feeling can come from a high-glycemic load, insulin resistance, inadequate sleep patterns or sleep apnea, or low testosterone levels, specifically during andropause or menopause. The antidote, he suggests, is eating small and frequent meals that are composed of proteins and complex low-glycemic carbohydrates and to correct any underlying medical problems.

I didn't know it back then. The food was controlling my moods and energy levels. Now when I'm facing down a delicious-looking cake, I ask myself, "How will it make me feel?" I am clear on the answer: It will taste heavenly going down but will make me feel downright icky, depressed, and bogged down afterward! I don't *ever* want to feel that way again. The Pavlovian desire to feel good and energetic makes it impossible for me to eat the way I used to.

This is extreme, but it works. I carry around a "before" picture to show people while they chow down on the bread and I sip my mineral water and eat a salad with cheese or walnuts. My circle of friends has changed, too. The people in my life tend to think more like me. There aren't a lot of us out there, but if you look hard enough, you can see past the "donut eaters."

I have been to Overeaters Anonymous and Weight Watchers, and I have tried everything from the grapefruit diet to Atkins to shed weight. All diets seem to work for a bit. And then comes the moment when you are tempted and you have "just one" cookie or brownie, one taste of whatever . . . and then just one more. Anyone who has dieted endlessly knows the scene. I realized that, for me, "moderation" was not an option. I had to take a hard line. Small doses of anything sugary would set me off.

And support, while it was comforting, was not something I could sustain. Real life didn't give me the luxury of taking time for bitch sessions. I didn't need to confess my indiscretions of the week or commiserate with others. I found that, for me, exercising in my spare time was a lot more productive.

IT'S ALL ABOUT ENERGY

My "diet," if you will, was an evolution. I read up on supplements. I spoke to nutritionists, doctors, nurses, and personal trainers. I began with a few supplements. What a pain in the neck to remember to take pills each day! But I made it routine and slipped into the mode. Supplements didn't kick in right away, but eventually they seemed to take effect. My cravings were less intense. That was step one. Then I removed sugar from my diet. It's astonishing how much sugar the average American eats without even realizing it! In doing so, I boosted my energy, which enabled me to work out more. In turn, this helped me lose weight and look better. The cycle is fueled by energy; the energy is fueled by what I ingest. Calcium and glucosamine keep my bones and joints strong so I can stay in motion and use that energy, maximizing my physical potential. The omegas appear to boost my mood.

Figuring out what to take and in what doses was a trial-and-error process for me. I tried many formulations that gave me headaches and didn't work for me. I spent a lot of money on pills that didn't seem to work. But I am a believer in learning and trying and in taking responsibility for my own health. Eventually a routine was born.

My supplement regimen is not about a magic weight-loss pill, but rather, it is designed to tone my mind. I have found that once I am feeling energetic and happy, my body tends to follow suit. Energy leads to strength and keeps me from falling into "couch potato" mode.

Nowadays, I travel with pills and potions. My day begins with supplements. Lots of them. But before I share my experiences, I would like to qualify them because I am not interested in pushing pills or potions. I can only share anecdotally what has worked for me and give you the theory behind why it may be working. I am no expert in nutrition, just someone who stumbled onto something that appears to work for me.

Before you take supplements, you should research them, ask lots of questions, and consult a physician. You should also find out which companies are known to have pure assays and better products. And you may want to investigate the inert ingredients in case you are allergic to some of the additives. Unlike pharmaceuticals, nutraceuticals are not closely monitored as medications but, rather, as foods. I do not endorse any one product over another. Having worked behind the scenes as a publicist for many nutraceutical companies, I have found that there is a strong caveat emptor factor in deciding which product to use. Many are repackaged and most are marked up outrageously. Learn about the nutraceuticals. Learn about the companies selling them. Ask about the purity of the particular formulation that you think might benefit you. Find out just what you are ingesting before you buy any over-the-counter nutraceuticals. Nutraceuticals are costly and generally not reimbursable by insurance companies. Don't believe outrageous claims, but do look at the research that has been done. Research interactions and contraindications to medications you take. Then make your choices, give them enough time to take effect, and if something isn't working, throw it away!

That said, I have found that these formulations work for me.

- **L-Carnitine and Co-Enzyme Q10** (A.M.) L-Carnitine is a compound said to be critical in transporting fatty acids into the cell mitochondria for energy production. It has been researched in the areas of cardiovascular diseases, physical performance enhancement, kidney function, and Alzheimer's disease and age-related senility. CoQ10 also improves energy production and acts as an antioxidant. Its effects are said to address prevention and treatment of cardiovascular disease and cancer. As an antioxidant, it specifically targets lipid peroxidation (yep, that means it affects fat cells).

It preserves the activity of vitamin E and helps prevent damage to lipid membranes and plasma lipids. CoQ10 works in concert with L-Carnitine.

- **Calcium with Magnesium** (A.M. and before bedtime, too) An adequate intake of daily dietary calcium is said to help control heart rate, blood clotting, muscle contraction, and more. Magnesium is said to help facilitate enzymatic reactions in the human body, contributing to the production of cardiovascular functions and the production and synthesis of energy. It also enhances the absorption of calcium and works hand in hand with calcium to contract muscles and relax them, as well as relax and calm nerves.

- **Glucosamine with Chondroitin Sulfate** (also in the A.M. and P.M.) Glucosamine is said to be an elemental building block required for biosynthesis of connective tissue, such as the cartilage found in joints. Chondroitin sulfate has been shown to be effective in the repair and restoration of cartilaginous tissue.

- **Slimmin' Up** (A.M.) This nutrient-rich herbal formula is said to reduce hunger and increase one's sense of energy.

- **Reneu** (A.M.) Designed to help cleanse and detoxify the intestinal system. A cleaner intestinal system helps enhance the absorption of vitamins, minerals, and herbal extracts, thereby optimizing weight management.

- **Omega-3 Fish Oil Pills and Ground Flaxseed** (A.M.) This combination of essential fatty acids is said to address conditions ranging from immune disorders, neural imbalances, joint problems, cancer, inflammation, kidney function, AIDS, and cardiovascular disease. They function as components of nerve cells, cell membranes, and hormone-like substances called prostaglandins.

- **Green Tea**—As much as I can chug all day.

I start each day with a shake—a breakfast protein drink comprising isolated soy proteins and whey. The one I choose is part of the Body FX program, made with fructose so it starts me in the right direction, not spiking my sugar. I've experimented with a lot of breakfasts, but since I try to spend some time after breakfast doing a cardio workout, I need something that will give me energy without the sluggish feeling that sugars and carbs seem to produce. I add ground flaxseed and sometimes a grain packaged as Salba to boost the omega-3s in the shake.

I have tried eating carbs before workouts, but it slows me down and makes me less energetic while I exercise. Protein is what my body craves while I am working to burn calories.

TIP

Test the waters. Become more aware of how food influences your mood and energy level. Keep a "food-mood diary" and note how you feel after eating various foods. You may begin to see correlations between high-protein or high-carb meals and your own energy level. Adjust your food balance and note changes (if any) before and after exercise.

DISCIPLINE

For me, the road to The Thin Club began with discipline and substitutions. I substituted sugar-free sweets, nuts, or high-fiber, low-sugar fruits (in careful moderation) when I needed a snack. Instead of sitting in front of the television, I found things to do that kept me active. I loathed being a participant and not a spectator. These days, if I do choose to watch TV, I exercise at the same time. My stability ball has become my ottoman. A Body Wedge stands in my living room, as do some free weights, reminding me that even relaxation and downtime don't have to be an excuse to vegetate. Even my children will pick up the free weights while they are watching television. It sure beats leaving a bowl of chips in the center of the table for them.

Just as the supplements gave me energy, as I began to eat more protein and less starchy carbs, I developed more energy. It was a self-perpetuating cycle. Less sugar meant more energy, which translated into the desire for more activity, which of course meant better results in weight loss and a more toned body. And looking in the mirror and seeing sleek muscle tone makes me want to continue eating healthy.

These days I confine myself to a mere bite of dessert if I really hanker to taste something special, but I'm more likely to treat myself to a side order of spinach or an extra helping of fish. Food is no longer a reward—it is fuel. It's fuel that my body needs to give me the energy to get through my day, to care for my children, to do my work. It's food that, if taken in the wrong amounts or comprising the wrong ingredients, will now give me a headache, a bloaty feeling, and a dry mouth at night.

Whereas my days used to be centered on what to eat,

what to make for dinner, which bakery in my neighborhood to go to for the best chocolate pudding pie or cream
cake (and I would drive miles for the right cream cake),
now I just grab a protein bar or shake; I'd rather get my
work done so I can hit the gym.

TIP

*Focus on the "good" carbs like nuts and berries and
avoid the sugar fixes.* Sugar is the culprit in obesity.
For some reason nature made the taste of sugar seduc-
tive. Even too much fruit can cause an overabundance
of sugar and can drag you into low energy and a lack-
luster mood.

While support groups did not work for me, many find
that working with buddies is beneficial. As you will see in
Chapter 8 on "Friends and Foes," not all weight-loss buddies are going to have your best interests at heart. Weight-
loss programs are frequently in business to make money,
and the way they make money is by repeat (translated to
yo-yo) business. Keeping someone in The Thin Club is certainly not going to fill their coffers. This paradox turned
me off to many of the popular diet groups that I tried over
the years.

My transition has been largely in my mind. Life is no
longer all about food. And I'm not the only one who
has lost weight and got trim in the process. My children are reaping the benefits of diet and exercise, too.
Dinner for them is frequently salad, fish or chicken, and a
sweet potato or sushi made with brown rice or whole
wheat pasta (they can have more of that since they are

able to process the sugar and carbs; I limit my carb portions).

Can anyone do what I've done? I totally believe they can. In fact, as you read my story, you will understand why I became heavy and why food became such a focus for me. My life was more extreme than many, but everyone has challenges. And, yes, it is possible for anyone to seize control of her or his life and care for herself or himself, no matter how dysfunctional things are.

The key to success is self-analysis, self-actualization, putting food in its proper perspective, finding exercise that thrills you and makes you look forward to it, changing your cupboard and refrigerator, but most of all, changing your mindset. So many of us are victims by nature. We are victims of our circumstances, our lifestyle, body type, intelligence level, career or lack of career. But nobody should ever be the victim of a candy bar or supersize french fries. Being a victim is largely a function of perception. And stepping out of victim mode is the secret to succeeding, not just in weight loss but also in life, in the workplace—you name it! Victim mentality is something that we can and *should* control. And once you learn to control that, you may be surprised at how other things fall into place as well.

ON THE WAY DOWN

You are getting sleeeeeepy! No, hypnosis won't make you cluck like a chicken. Rosie Schulman, Dr. Harold Schulman's wife and a registered nurse, helped me jump-start my diet with it. Rosie was the person who looked at me even when I was still a good sixty pounds overweight and said I was an athlete. An athlete? Since my athletic activities until that point had been confined to opening and shutting the refrigerator door, I thought she was crazy. Now as I hop to and from Pilates, kickboxing, and jujitsu in my spandex yoga clothes, Rosie and I laugh at my late-blooming athletic prowess. She was right, and perhaps the very suggestion, hypnotic or not, was what helped set my course.

As I began to lose weight, issues started to crop up— issues that I realized, if not addressed, could impede or, worse, affect my overall success. I didn't try hypnosis to lose weight but, rather, to address some of these issues and to learn to isolate and combat the messages that came from years of reinforced negative behavior patterns. An early problem for me was the issue of strength and power.

As I proceeded downscale, I realized that I had a history of power struggles, beginning with my parents and later with my husband, and even with work colleagues and my own children. I recognized that I found myself frequently feeling victimized by these negative feelings. Power and weight seemed somehow related. My excess weight was insulation—protection; in some ways it made me feel safe, but in other ways I felt helpless. I needed strength. I told Rosie. We talked about the issues of safety, power, and strength and then she put me under. Putting me in a state of total relaxation, she helped me get in touch with the negative feelings that were crippling me and keeping me from achieving my goals—both on the scale and off of it. An hour later I felt strong, ready to face down any cream pie, extra helping, lazy-bones inclination that was keeping me from the gym, as well as being an impediment to my success. I left with a surge of energy, and the energy got stronger with time.

A few months later I found the strength to leave my marriage—one that had been riddled with physical and emotional abuse for twenty-two years. I reclaimed my children, boosted my business to support my family, moved out of my home, and became a powerful new person. Hypnosis certainly wasn't the only factor, but it was a large piece of the puzzle that helped me piece my life back together.

MY JOURNEY DOWNSCALE

The First Fifteen Pounds

Everyone starts a diet with a new sense of resolve and a little trepidation. I certainly did. I remember going to the doctor after my angiogram and telling him that I had resolved to lose weight. "What should I do?" I asked him.

He looked at me, clueless. "You've been on diets before," he said. "You know the drill . . . lots of cottage cheese and walk around a lot. Or try Weight Watchers." I tried Weight Watchers. I used their online journaling system. And it helped for a while. The first fifteen pounds were the most important to me. They were the pounds that propelled me into my initial excitement phase. They were also the ones that "detoxed" my body from the things that made me fat. Initially, I went on a regular program. It worked. I lost weight. Once a week I would reward myself with some sugary treat. It made me feel like I was cheating, but I still lost weight.

While the psychological motivation was loud and clear during this phase, I had trouble with cravings. My body wanted to go back to status quo—and the foods I craved were precisely the ones I needed to cut out completely from my diet. My diet buddies were very important to me at this stage of the game. I found myself on the phone with them constantly, feeling attacked by Girl Scout cookies, bread, pasta—you name it. It seemed that these seducers were everywhere.

I began my diet with a motivational shopping trip at Catherine's, a large-size clothing store. Yes, I shopped before I even lost a single pound, and if you are in the beginning phase of a weight loss, so should you! I bought myself a few items and tried to avoid my bulging reflection in the dressing-room mirror. It made me want to run to the nearest Carvel for a double-size hot fudge sundae! Thanks to my cell phone and a little help (OK, a *lot* of help) from my friends, I managed to resist the temptations.

The Latent Phase
After I was fifteen pounds down, the scale was getting a tad closer to 200 pounds. Would I ever get below that number? I was hopeful, but I still felt like a tank. This phase is when the diet becomes more challenging and when people typically start losing their motivation. Even though my clothes were starting to get a bit looser, I was still over a size 20 and knew I was a long way from ever seeing my way out of the plus-size shops.

I watched the pounds go up and down in a typical weight-loss pattern. Sometimes I gained a pound or two, then the next week I'd lose three. I tried to stick to my diet. The scale was a depressing reminder. Just as I would wake up feeling "extra-skinny," I'd hop on the scale and realize that I had actually gained a pound! Now, what was that all about? Why bother with this stupid diet?

I was not quite ready to exercise, but I began to have the energy to think about it. I was in the middle of writing a book and was beginning to think about promoting it. I thought about appearing on *Oprah* someday to talk about my book. I wanted to go on TV. The camera adds ten pounds, maybe the ten pounds I had just lost. I had been on *Oprah* when I wrote my first book, and my big, round face had taken up the whole TV screen. All I saw back then was my double chin and jowls, hideously jiggling up and down as I commented, albeit intelligently, on the topic. I didn't want to be all chin and jowls again. That kept me motivated. I broke the 200-pound barrier.

Eureka!

This is the phase when you begin to reap the fruits of your long labor and you start to see noticeable results. Suddenly my fat clothes were truly "fat clothes." Even belts couldn't save me from the inevitable. I was thin—well, thinner. I needed new clothes. I was starting to look good. Really good. I was also scared. Really scared. Even though I still had many pounds to go to get anywhere near my goal, my body was beginning to reflect the fruits of my diet. I was beginning to get attention. I didn't know how to negotiate this new scrutiny. It had been years since anyone had scrutinized my body. People were noticing the weight loss. This is the point where I started to yo-yo. I fudged just a little bit on my diet and gained weight back.

We had recently moved and I was baking and cooking to impress the neighbors. I wanted to be a success. Food was something I was "good at." You can't bake and cook without tasting, can you? I gained a few pounds at first, then a few more. One day, while sitting in a beauty parlor, I complained to the hairstylist about my yo-yo plight. He introduced me to Rosie. Rosie looked me over from head to toe. She explained to me that perhaps it wasn't what I was eating or how much—perhaps it was something more. She offered to hypnotize me.

I thought she was nuts. But ever open to new ideas, I made an appointment with Rosie and shortly thereafter found myself sitting in a darkened room, listening to the sound of waves crashing upon the shore. It felt like a garage door was slamming down when I went under. My muscles were totally relaxed. My mouth slackened, I drooled a bit, and my eyes teared. I didn't move to wipe my face. I listened to Rosie's voice, soft and slow. In that room, Rosie told me that I was strong, I was athletic, I had the strength and power to do anything I wanted to do. It went beyond weight loss. Strength permeated my being. I was in a deep state of consciousness. I prayed for control. I found it and resisted the Samoa Girl Scout cookies.

I was back in charge and began my downward journey once more. I was determined to make it happen for good this time. I took some money I had earned in an insurance settlement and invested in a series of Pilates classes with a personal trainer. It was gentle exercise and slowly I began to regain my confidence. I could exercise. It felt good—I was a little sore afterward but it was a good kind of sore. I kept going. I was developing more energy every day, and eventually I added cardiovascular activity to my workout. As I exercised, I became more hungry. I could eat more . . . or so I thought. Being an athlete required a new approach to my weight-loss program.

The Plateau

This was probably the most delicate and difficult phase for me. I was depriving myself of all the foods I had once loved and exercising hard, yet if I was lucky I dropped a half a pound. Frustration set in as I kept "being good" and yet, somehow, the scale didn't move. It could have sent me straight to the dessert table; instead, I called Rosie. She advised me to try a new, low-glycemic approach: cut the sugar and balance the proteins with high-fiber carbs. She was my guru. I listened and was back in the saddle again. "You're an athlete," she reminded me. An athlete can surely shake up her exercise routine, I figured. So I did. I began to cross-train, adding weights to the treadmill and belly dancing to the Pilates. The pounds and dress sizes were dropping again.

Metamorphosis Realized

So when will I ever really believe I'm thin? Sometimes I do; much of the time I don't. But somewhere along the line, I stopped weighing myself obsessively whenever I "broke" my diet. When I finally learned to balance eating too large a portion with an extra ten minutes on the treadmill, and I recognized that eating an extra piece of sweet potato didn't mean I could give myself permission to eat an entire cream pie for dessert, I knew I had begun to accept myself as a person who will never again be a fat girl. It was a slow but steady change—the ultimate "change of life."

I began to buy clothes that were hip, flashy, even sexy. It was during this phase that I finally learned that I was indeed perceived as thin by the rest of the world (even when I felt that I had yet another ten pounds to lose) and I began to fight the rest of the brain battles that go along with joining The Thin Club (to be enumerated in this book). I finished writing my last book with the newfound realization that I was not a victim. And I realized that the only saboteur and victimizer around was myself. I seized control, a victim no longer. I never did make it back onto *Oprah,* but I have been on television many times since; after a few blinks, I realized that my chin no longer jiggles and I look a whole lot slimmer than I thought I would look. I still saw the fat girl, but she wasn't quite "as fat." And that to me was the day I let the world know: I've joined The Thin Club! It's a membership I'm proud of and one that I've earned.

It hasn't always been an easy road to follow, and a day will not go by when I don't consider carefully the choice between eating something or not, of skipping an exercise session or not, and of risking a larger dress size or not. I have become more aware of the choices, in both public and private. And in the immortal words of Yogi Berra, "It ain't over till it's over." Toning your mind is a never-ending commitment.

PART ONE

WHAT IF THE WEIGHT COMES BACK?

How to Handle

the Most Common

Concerns and Fears

Following

Weight Loss

TWO

FEAR OF THE FAT COMING BACK

THE HOLIDAYS ARE HERE. AND HOORAY! VISIONS OF sugarplums no longer tempt me. Well, not *that* much anymore. But I have been so busy with holiday preparations—taking care of everyone else—that I have been remiss in my exercise regime. And I'd be a liar if I didn't say that I'm experiencing high anxiety. Not about preparing the perfect pumpkin pie; rather, it's about the possibility of accumulating excess holiday poundage. I know, practically speaking, that I should be making time for exercise and that less exercise means I have to adjust my caloric intake. But the stress of preparing, and the ups and downs of everyday living as a single working mother with umpteen daily challenges, is putting me in a no-exercise, heavy-duty eating mode.

"WHAT IF . . . !"

The worst stressor of all are the "What ifs." What if this temporary lapse results in the return of the weight? Some of the weight? All of the weight? What if I don't resume my exercise routine when I finally can? What if I do and I can't get up to speed at my regular pace? What if my nice sexy muscles turn mushy again? What if my clothes start feeling tight at the waist? What if I have to buy fat clothes again? What if people start noticing the love handles I'm starting to see? Are they real or imagined?

I'm enjoying a special dinner with my family. I reach for a cookie. It wasn't nearly as good as I thought it would be. I have another. And then I'm gripped by the ridiculous desire to run to the nearest scale or mirror to see the results of my errant behavior. Should I try starvation? I know better than that! It doesn't work and only makes me hungrier in the long run. I feel more vulnerable now than I have in ages. The list of "I won't ever touch" food items is enormous for me. Before the weight loss, I worried, "What if I can never lose this weight?" Now that it's gone, I wonder, "What if the weight comes back?"

I've become used to being svelte. I love the attention I get when I whip out my fat photos and people squint and hold them up—in complete disbelief that I ever could have looked like that. The thought of going back in the up direction is paralyzing! I've become accustomed to seeing myself as a success. If I put on weight—even a few pounds—I will feel like a failure again. I'm so scared.

I resolve to take not a single bite of something questionable. I vow to watch the volume of food and to limit my intake of nuts, protein, and other food that I'm "allowed." But most of all, I promise myself to keep exercising. And to find outlets other than food for whatever is driving me to eat.

THE WILLPOWER CONUNDRUM

Many people have lost weight before, only to have it return (and sometimes gain more), and others have struggled so much to lose weight that they feel it is too good to be true when it actually happens. There are so many worries that can sabotage your weight-loss strength:

- What if I lose my willpower?
- What if I gain all my weight back and more?

Unfortunately, these types of thoughts lead to anxiety and an increased probability that the weight loss will *not* be sustained. It is very difficult to accept and enjoy your post-diet body when you are constantly wondering how long it will last. The fear of regaining the weight is one of the biggest factors in whether or not you do regain the weight. It prevents you from truly enjoying the weight loss, and it makes it more likely that you'll regain the weight—not a good combination. This chapter is about how to overcome those fears and worries.

WHY YOUR FEAR COMES TRUE

When Larina meets new people and says that she helps people to lose weight and keep it off, she hears all kinds of stories. A common response is, "I recently lost thirty pounds! It feels great but I'm so nervous that I'll gain it back!" If you have this fear, you are not alone. In fact, there are few people (if any) who have lost a substantial amount of weight and have *not* worried about gaining it back.

These fears make a lot of sense. First, they're grounded in reality because most of those who lose weight *do* regain the weight within a few years. Second, you worked very hard, and it's painful to think about having to go through the whole process again. Third, sometimes the things you think about and fear are the things that you consciously or unconsciously make come true. Let's go through these ideas one by one.

THE REAL STORY ABOUT WEIGHT REGAIN

We hate to be the bearer of bad news, but the fear of weight coming back has a strong basis to it. Research shows that most people are unable to keep lost weight off. Most people regain the weight within three years. We know—you're thinking this book is being written to help you stop worrying and now we are giving you reason to worry! One of the first steps to overcoming a fear is to understand whether the fear is logical or not. Well, the fear of weight regain is logical. *But,* here's the good news. Whether or not you actually regain the weight is something that's within your control. It's not as if you are afraid of the stock market crashing, something which you really can't control. The only one who's in charge of whether or not the fear comes true is *you*! Of course, that puts some pressure on you, but it's also very empowering. And once you overcome your fears, you are in a much better position to make sure the weight regain does not happen.

TIP

Recognize your worries. The first step in overcoming weight-gain anxieties is to see when and where they come up. Is it before you go out to dinner? When you shop for clothes or food? Write these worries down and decide whether they are logical or not. A logical worry is one that makes sense given the circumstances, such as knowing you are likely to be confronted with a trigger food or trigger situation, as opposed to a random fear. If the worries seem random, dismiss them. Read on, we'll tell you how.

THE CONFIDENCE KILLER

One of the big reasons that your fears about the weight's coming back are so harmful to you is that they zap your confidence. These fears make it hard to enjoy the weight loss that you worked hard for and deserve to celebrate. No matter how you lost your weight, whether through diet, exercise, or surgery, it was a challenge and it would be great if you could enjoy it. Once the worrying cycle starts, you lose your positive feelings and your confidence. It is difficult if not impossible to be anxious and confident at the same time.

What one quality do you think is extremely important in losing the fat and keeping it off? If you guessed confidence, you are absolutely right! If you're not confident in your abilities, who will be? Who will cheer you on and help you get through all those difficult decision points about what food to select? Who will tell you that you can do it even thought it's tough? Who will keep you motivated and inspired to stay on track even in the face of major enticement?

You need to be able to do these things for yourself. The ability to cheerlead yourself helps you to stay on track and keeps you inspired, motivated, and happy. Without confidence, it's tough to keep a healthy lifestyle in a world of constant temptations.

THE SELF-FULFILLING PROPHECY

Have you ever heard about a self-fulfilling prophecy? This is one of Larina's favorite concepts in psychology because it comes up in all aspects of life. It means that you create your own reality based on what you expect to happen. One of Larina's quotes on this topic is, "The thing that you believe is the very thing that you become." She believes that the idiom "You are what you eat" is less true than what she likes to remind clients: "You are what you see." If you still see yourself as weak, incapable, and fat, that is likely what will occur, even if you're now thin.

In an interesting study, researchers led men to believe that a woman they were about to speak with on the phone was attractive or unattractive. In reality, there was no difference in attractiveness between the women. When men believed the women were attractive, they spoke to them differently and more positively. The women responded favorably to the way these men talked with them. Independent raters listened to the conversations and rated the conversations. They found that the women who spoke with the men who thought they were talking to an attractive woman were more likeable, sociable, and attractive. So the men actually created more attractive women when they thought the woman was attractive!

If you believe that you will be fat again, there's a good chance that you will be. If you allow your fear to take over and sap your strength, the fear will probably win. If you don't fight your worries and work on disproving them, they can take over and come true. When you learn how to effectively handle these fears, you can control them. They are less likely to keep you in a constant state of anxiety. They are less likely to come true. Here's how . . .

A THIN CLUB MEMBER WEIGHS IN
Stacey Johnson (age thirty-four, Phoenix, Arizona) has been successful with losing weight and keeping it off by changing her food habits and exercising regularly. Stacey was open to making lifestyle changes despite her concern that nothing would work, based on her past experience of going up and down on the scale. She proved to herself that

she *can* do things that she never thought she could do. Stacey says:

> I pay attention to what's on my plate and my portion. And I drink lots of water. I listen to how I feel when I'm eating—if I'm eating too quickly, I slow down. If I'm getting full, I stop. If I'm running low on energy and need a snack, I have a snack. I'm learning to trust myself and respond accordingly and modify my eating to fit when I'm hungry. This helps me to even out the portion sizes of my meals and snacks.
>
> So much has changed. I wear color now! I used to always be in black and navy and now I wear all the colors. I've learned that I can have control and eat smaller portions. I don't deprive myself and don't overdo it like I used to. I even eat chocolate regularly. It's been a journey for me—after spending so many years back and forth—and it's going great!

Stacey became pregnant with her second child and was thrilled, but nervous about packing the pounds back on. During her first pregnancy, she admits that she used it as an excuse to eat for two or three or four. When she became pregnant with her second child, she worried about whether she'd be able to maintain the eating habits that helped her lose the weight. About staying in The Thin Club even during pregnancy, Stacey says:

> The hardest part for me has been accepting that I'm going to gain weight. I was nervous that it would be too much weight, but I actually found that because of my healthy lifestyle, I continued to lose weight initially and then gained because of the pregnancy, not because of my

*unhealthy eating habits. It's been fun to wear these preg-
nancy clothes—the ones I couldn't wear during my first
pregnancy.*

*I was nervous about getting pregnant because I was
still working on weight loss and much of the first trimester,
I worried that I'd gain all the weight back. It was a struggle for me emotionally. My doctors let me know that it was
OK to gain slowly and not gain too much weight during
the pregnancy. Hearing this was a relief. My doctor didn't
want me to diet and lose much, but it was great to know
that it's healthy to maintain the weight or gain very gradually by eating well-balanced, healthy foods and exercising.*

*Pregnancy is a different experience for me now because
before I was concerned that people looked at what I ate in
a negative, judgmental way. I thought they'd be thinking
about how much I ate and how unhealthy it was. Now,
I'm eating healthy foods in the right-sized portions and
people make comments like, "you need to eat more." It actually makes me smile because I know I'm in control and
doing the right thing and being healthy. It's empowering to
know that people's comments and judgments don't negatively impact me anymore—people can judge either way
but it doesn't have to bother you.*

*Focusing on my plan after the baby keeps me moti-
vated. Setting short-term goals for how much weight to lose
before returning to work is helpful. Because I was able to
lose weight and keep it off for a long time before this pregnancy, I'm confident that I can take it off—I've done it before and can do it again. And it will be easier because I
didn't revert back to old eating habits and gain a lot of
weight since I've continued my healthy lifestyle.*

*This time I want to have pictures of me pregnant. Now,
I'm proud of it. Last time I felt big, fat, and ugly and*

wanted to hide. I wasn't eating well or exercisi
gaining weight where I should because of the
and I want to remember it. People complime
it makes me feel good and more inclined to i
brace it.

HOW TO QUELL FOOD ANXIETIES

Here are some steps to overcome your fear and anxieties. Try each of these strategies separately and see which ones work for you. If one doesn't work, keep practicing it, since it's likely to help you eventually, but it can take some time and practice.

THE ART OF ACCEPTANCE

In overcoming anxiety about food (or any anxiety, for that matter), one of the fundamental first steps is to accept it. It may sound weird since it's also important to fight your fears, but fighting and accepting are two opposite things. But you can do both. In order to beat it, you must first join it.

Recognizing the presence of your fears and worries is crucial. Once you know what they are, you can accept their presence. As discussed, it makes a lot of sense that you would have your worries, so don't judge yourself for having them. Don't think of yourself as weak or incompetent, or in trouble because you're worried about regaining the weight you lost. Everybody has these worries! They are completely normal and it would be strange if you never had them. Instead, accept that these worries are natural.

Sometimes the mere art of accepting worries is enough to make them go away. The cycle of anxiety is fueled by

g to fight it off. If you have a worry and you keep push-
ng it down, it keeps popping back up. It is like bouncing a
ball. If you keep hitting it down, it keeps bouncing back
up. If, on the other hand, you don't hit it down, it will keep
bouncing for a few seconds, but with each bounce it loses
momentum and soon it will stop bouncing.

This idea of handling worries is a strange one because
the natural response is to fight them away and push them
down. Do the opposite. The first step is to bring them to
the surface and know what you're really afraid of. Then,
stop pushing them away. As a result, they should naturally
calm down and become less intense.

TIP

Practice accepting anxiety. Everytime you notice a
worry or fear come along, tell yourself that it has a right
to be there. Don't judge yourself for having it or overly
react to it. Picture that you put the worry on a cloud and
let it sit there, and eventually it will get carried away with
the wind.

MAINTAINING THE PERSPECTIVE

Once you know what your fears truly are, you'll be able to
put them into perspective. Ask yourself:

- Are you nervous that you'll gain weight back and
  disappoint your spouse or significant other?
- Are you afraid of feeling like a failure?
- Does the idea that you'll be deprived forever haunt
  you?
- Do you worry that something stressful will happen
  and you'll turn to eating?

- What are you really afraid of?
- What's the worst fear?

Once you can answer these questions you can gain perspective over the worry. Anxious thoughts are characterized by all or none thinking. This means that you are more likely to think in black or white. You think that you either can do it or you'll fail; that once you start eating an "off-limits" food you'll succumb to eating tons of it every day; that you are eating "well" or "horribly." It's one extreme or another.

When you are wrapped up in an emotion such as anxiety, you get tunnel vision. You become so focused on your fear that you forget about everything else around you. You may sit in front of a buffet table at a party worrying that you will dive in at any point in time. In the midst of that fear and tunnel vision, you forget about all the things you can do to handle the situation. You can walk to another part of the room. You can talk to a friend. You can hold something in your hand or chew gum to keep you from eating. You can use your newfound knowledge about food to make the right choices, like fat-burning red pepper sans the fattening dip. There are tons of things you can do, but you lose perspective when you're caught in the moment of fear. Gain perspective by thinking through your fears rationally. Write them down. Talk to a friend or a professional about them. Distance yourself from them and look at them objectively as someone else would.

Now you can begin to gain perspective over the fear and learn that it isn't necessarily true. One of the best ways to gain perspective is to make the fear less black or white. Question it. Is it really true that you'll gain all your weight back once you start eating a certain food? Must you be either deprived or gluttonous? Recognize the gray areas.

In reality, weight is regained pound by pound. The fear would have you think that you'll wake up fat one morning. Things are not as black or white as the fear would have you believe they are. When you see the gray areas, you learn that you can intervene during those times. If you've gained back five pounds, you can do something about it and get back on track. Now is the time to start taking action to disprove the fears.

TIP

Fill in the gray areas. When you notice an all-or-nothing type of thought pop into your mind, decide to look for alternative explanations. Ask yourself, "What are some other possibilities that could explain this situation or some other outcomes that could occur?" This process of challenging your thoughts will help prevent tunnel vision and will give you a broader perspective on the situation. If you have difficulty doing this at first, get others to help you. Call an objective friend, or join a support group.

DISPROVING YOUR FEARS

The best way to teach yourself not to worry is to prove to yourself that worries are often wrong. How many times have you worried about something, only to find out that it didn't come true? This is the futility of worry.

Yes, You *Can* Eat Just One!

This is where you get to have some fun talking back to your fears and showing them that they needn't bug you. The way to do this is to try to do the thing that you're afraid of. For instance, if you're worried that you'll feel deprived forever, you can have a small piece of chocolate and disprove the idea that you're totally deprived. If you're afraid that you could never eat another french fry without gorging on them, eat a fry.

The best way to set up these little experiments is to do them in a way that helps yourself win. Remember, you are trying to prove the fear wrong, so you should do whatever you can to give yourself the advantage. For example, go out to lunch with a friend and have her save you a single french fry. Eat the fry right before you leave so you can't order more fries. (You're trying to stack the deck in your favor so that you won't eat tons of fries.) When you have the one fry, you teach the fear that it is often wrong and you can handle it.

Even if your fear comes true, you can ask yourself how many times it *hasn't* come true. If it came true one time out of one hundred times that you worried about it, then it is only 1 percent likely to come true. This probably isn't as bad as you thought. In this process, you're taking the power out of the fear. You gain the power back by taking the matter into your own hands. You are empowered when you actively address it. You are further empowered when you work to disprove it.

TIP

Talk to yourself as you'd talk to a child. If a child says, "I can't do that!" you would provide him or her encouragement to try it out anyway. You may say, "You never know unless you try" or "Why not try and find out?" If the kid was afraid to do something, you'd set up the situation so the child would have a positive experience. You'd select a manageable situation that you know the boy or girl could handle. Do the same for yourself. Don't sit down with a pint of ice cream. Instead, go to a frozen yogurt store and get a small portion-controlled cup or a sugar-free dessert.

A PICTURE IS WORTH . . .

I love my camera. Not because the camera loves me—it does not. When I take a photo (and now it is so easy with digital cameras that upload pictures to your computer screen!) I can see every bulge in my midsection, every roll of back fat, loose skin on my arms—it is undeniable! And why do I love seeing the bulges? Because somehow, I have developed "mirror blindness." When I stand in front of the mirror I can pose a certain way, catch my best angles, and fool myself into thinking that yes, I *can* skip the kickboxing class or eat that piece of bread that is calling my name. A photograph doesn't cut me the same slack.

Maybe the camera does add ten pounds, but that is just the kick in the pants I need to keep me on the straight and narrow. So I photograph myself often (it's great to keep current photos available online to send friends, relatives, and, if you're single, dating sites), and I wear clothes that cling, not clothes that hide (jackets, bulky sweaters, etc.). It's just another tool to train my mind to cut through the denial mechanisms and see what others see when they look at me.

TIP

Use your camera. The camera can help give you an objective look at how others see you and the photos can keep you motivated. Take a picture of yourself when you think you look great and carry it around with you. This will keep you inspired to keep looking like that or to work on looking like that with a bit more toning and exercise.

PUTTING THESE STEPS TOGETHER

OK, let's put together the steps to overcoming your fear of the fat coming back. First, recognize your fears. Write them down. Become aware of them. It is important that you know exactly what you are really afraid of. A vague understanding of the fear is not enough. Try to figure out the underlying biggest fear.

Next, accept the worries. Imagine that your fear is a helium-filled balloon in the room. If you keep pushing it down, it'll keep popping up. Why not let it float up to the ceiling and leave you alone?

Now, you have a new perspective on the fear. When you look at the balloon from the bottom, you can study it and find ways to put a hole in it or untie the knot that keeps the air in it. You start to look for holes in the fear's argument. You help yourself to see that your fear is unlikely to come true. You realize that even if it did come true, which is unlikely, you could find ways to manage it.

At this point, you begin to actively challenge the fear by doing what you are afraid of in a safe, controlled situation. You learn that you can handle it. This is powerful. Using the idea of the balloon, if you let it float on your ceiling after accepting its presence, it would eventually lose the helium and come down. This is a fine strategy. But you can make it happen faster and more powerfully by letting the air out of the balloon. Each time you do something you are afraid of and learn that the consequences aren't disastrous, you take some air out of the balloon of fear.

TIP

Write a personal success story. Document all the obstacles and objections you confronted and how you overcame them. If you have a hard time giving yourself credit for your accomplishments, write the story in the third person, as if it's about someone else. You'll be better able to assess your strengths and successes. Read this story at least once a week to keep your mind "thin."

The more things you do to confront your fear, the more you build your confidence and the fear shrinks away. Keep in mind that you can use this process for fears that aren't related to weight and eating as well. The more you feel confident, in control, and empowered in your life in general, the more you will be able to manage your eating as well. By working on overcoming other fears and anxieties, you will be more able to overcome your fear of the fat's returning. The more practice you get using these strategies, the easier they will become and the more effective they will be. Try them and find out.

TIP

Remember that the point of becoming thin is to lead a healthy, enjoyable life. If you become paralyzed by fear and avoid every outing with friends, every dinner party, and every trip to the amusement park with kids, you'll be controlled by the fear and you will miss out on all the benefits of being in The Thin Club. Proceed with caution and planning, but do proceed with the activities that are intimidating but an important part of leading a balanced, happy life.

THREE

YOUR RELATIONSHIP WITH FOOD

Addressing the Hidden Meanings

SOME OF MY EARLIEST MEMORIES ARE OF FOOD fights! Not the *Animal House,* pie-flinging, gob-stuffed, splats-of-food-hitting-white-togas variety, but rather the "*Who* ate the donuts I bought for my class?" or the "*Why* did you eat that cookie? Don't you realize it may not be for you? What *were* you thinking?" kind.

I remember, at two years old, having my tear-filled screaming fits ended with a crumbly sugar cookie topped with a big green cherry, handed to me by the clerk at the Bergen Bake Shop in Newark. And although I was younger than three, I still recall Mr. Stimler, the butcher, smiling as he gave me a slice of salami—anything to keep me from flinging myself into a preschool tizzy on his sawdusted butcher-store floor. Food was a way of drying my tears, quelling my fears, and making me believe that while I may not be receiving the item or, more important, the emotion (probably love and affection) that I really craved, the taste of sweet, sour, salty, and spicy could placate, smooth over, and make me feel a little bit better about the world around me. For a little while.

A HISTORY OF ABUSE

I was emotionally abused as a child. There were ups and downs, and none of them made sense. There was yelling and screaming topped with teeth-gnashing angst. And there was sexual abuse. When I was four years old, I was sexually molested by four male teenagers. I didn't think about that incident until after I had lost the weight and begun taking Rape Escape classes. The flashbacks came fast and furious. I didn't use food to make them go away. I used my brain. I used my strength. I learned to defend myself.

I was a fat child with a pretty face. I became a chubby teenager with a pretty face. And the weight created a cycle: feel bad, eat, feel worse, eat more, look in the mirror, feel worse, eat still more.

"Doesn't your cousin have a beautiful figure?" my mother would snipe, ever so subtly. I heard the unspoken, "Not like you! Why can't *my* daughter have a lovely figure too?"

So by the time I met my husband, my self-esteem was thoroughly and completely submerged and destroyed. I was thrilled to find a man that seemed to love me. It meant I was lovable. On our second date, he looked at me adoringly and wondered aloud how I would look in a bikini. (You've *got* to be kidding, I thought, even though I was relatively thin—probably around 145 pounds at the time.) I told him I didn't feel comfortable with his talking like that about my body. In a fit of rage, he kicked me in the shins and at my insistence he took me home.

I refused to take his phone calls for two weeks. Then one day he slipped under the radar and managed to call me. I let myself listen to his apologies. He cried. He said he was sorry, and he wanted to make it up to me. I agreed to see him again. It was the beginning of an ongoing abusive relationship. And the more he abused me emotionally and physically, the more I punished myself with food. We married. I became the world's greatest cook. And I became the world's most fabulous eater. I cooked, I fed, and I ate. My world revolved around food. The relationship was a bittersweet one, in that it produced three sweet children but also a lot of pain and confusion.

It took me twenty-two years to garner the strength to leave. In one of my later hypnosis sessions with Rosie, I forgave my ex-husband for the pain he inflicted on me. It was not the same forgiveness I granted periodically during our marriage after one of his emotional rampages, in which I would swallow my anger, usually along with a pie or two; it was a more settled and complete forgiveness that allowed me to put the past behind me. I set myself free of the control issues that plagued me for so many years.

As a newlywed, I recall entertaining a colleague from work. She looked in horror at the heaping mounds of pasta on her plate. She was thin.

"I can't possibly eat all this," she said incredulously. I can, I thought, as I dug in.

By the time I became pregnant, I was already close to 160 pounds. Pregnant and scared, feeling weak and unprotected, I packed on the pounds. The weight gave me heft, not that I needed much to outweigh my husband, but it somehow made me feel stronger. Stronger—well, bigger— but in a way, weaker at the same time. I was weak-willed around food.

I learned to drown my tears in sweet whipped-cream cakes. Sometimes my husband would nag me about my weight. I ate more. Because, in some obscure way, food was something I could control; and by getting fatter and uglier, I was telling him that he would never really control me!

Oh, I did lose weight once before. I was twenty-eight years old and thin as a rail. And I galvanized my strength, got a new job, and was ready to leave the marriage. And then the magnitude of what I was doing—child in tow, taking control—hit me like a ton of bricks. I asked myself if I really thought any other man would be better. I answered myself with a no. And besides, I didn't want to be alone. Once again, my husband cried and swore things would change—he would change. I would never again wake up in the middle of the night with his hands around my neck. He even agreed to let me have that second child I'd been pining for. And so I got pregnant, and I let myself get fat again, and fatter and fatter. And by the time I was pregnant with my third child, and the abuse started up anew, I was about 200 pounds. Five years later, I was 225 pounds and growing, with no end in sight. But I was bigger than my husband and I felt protected by my girth! In some perverse way, being heavier made me feel stronger.

When my then eight-year-old was diagnosed with an illness, I was despondent. There seemed to be no way to cope with the diagnosis. I decided to write a book about surviving the situation. In doing so, I reached inward and found my strength. That success, combined with my health problems, was the closure I needed to confront the problems head on. I didn't want to be a martyr mom. I didn't want to be anyone's victim anymore.

I was ready to change. I was ready to be thin. I was ready to end the cycle of abuse and become a new person. After twenty-two years, I decided to start a new life.

USING FOOD TO COPE

It is common to eat as a way of dealing with a difficult past—or a difficult present. When people are emotionally, physically, or sexually neglected or abused, they often turn to food. Some people eat, consciously or unconsciously, to protect themselves and provide a barrier to the outside world and the people who may hurt them. When they lose the weight but have not dealt with past traumatic, difficult, or upsetting experiences, they may lack the confidence to truly keep the weight off.

While most obese and overweight individuals do not have a history of trauma, there are many who do. *Trauma* is typically defined as an actual or perceived threat to one's life or physical integrity, or that of someone else (such as by witnessing someone else being assaulted). You may have experienced trauma as defined here. Or you may have had experiences that were not classically traumatic but certainly were not positive. For example, perhaps you didn't grow up in a warm, nurturing environment. You may have been the victim of teasing, harassment, or abandonment as a child or an adult.

When you've had difficult life experiences, it makes sense that you would look for a solution to help you feel better. Food is a readily available, socially acceptable solution for many people. You can always get food; it is legal to purchase and eat; and you can easily overdose on food and get caught in a vicious cycle of stuffing down negative feelings with large amounts of food.

A PHYSICAL BARRIER

Sometimes people who have experienced abuse get heavy as a means of keeping people away from them or of feeling physically larger and having more of a presence. Some obese people, especially women, report that they gained weight after being sexually abused, as a way to protect or comfort themselves. Many women Larina and her colleagues have worked with state that they realized they were gaining weight but on some level they felt safer as they became heavier.

A layer of fat can feel like physical and psychological protection from a cruel world. It seems that people can't get to you as easily. You may feel physically more powerful as you increase the mass of your body and occupy more space in the world.

One patient who had survived a violent mugging once told Larina that she started to become increasingly anxious as she lost weight because she felt defenseless. As a smaller person, she felt like more of a target. She had worked hard for almost a year to lose weight, and she achieved her target weight loss. But the weight began creeping back because her fear increased as a thin woman, and she reverted to her old habit of using food to cope with anxiety. Until she dealt with the anxiety related to an assault she had experienced years before, she would be unable to live comfortably in a smaller body and would keep regaining lost weight.

Others add weight as a means of erecting a wall against society. Some reject the unattainable standards for beauty that are propagated in our society; in an act of rebellion, they eat more or revert to old eating habits. Others struggle between wanting to be seen as attractive and wanting to feel safe and not be noticed. This is a difficult tension to experience, and it becomes easy to drift to what feels easier or more comforting, which often involves eating and gaining weight.

There is a natural desire to be the best you can be, to appear attractive and feel good about yourself. Yet people who've experienced trauma often say that they want to blend in and be unnoticeable. If you are currently overweight or were overweight in the past, you may feel that people noticed you less as a fat person than when you're thin. For many, not being noticed translates to feeling safe and protected.

TIP

Create alternative ways to feel strong and empowered. Remember that protection by fat yields a false sense of security. Fat does not mean strong. There are many benefits to increasing your physical strength. Increased muscle mass can help you keep the weight off by increasing your resting metabolic rate, and it can help you feel strong in a smaller body. Take a self-defense class or pursue kickboxing or martial arts. Lift weights at the gym. Commit to doing push-ups and pull-ups every night.

THE FOOD BAND-AID

When you are violated, abandoned, or mistreated by people, it is natural to look for ways to nurture yourself. You probably know from your experience, or have heard, that food fills wounds that never heal. When you are injured, whether the injuries are physical or emotional, you look for ways to heal yourself. Unfortunately, using food to heal these wounds does not work. A wound needs to be cleaned out, exposed to the air, and allowed to heal on its own. If you constantly keep the wound covered up, it may not heal and also may get worse. It can become infected.

Food serves as a tight bandage over the wound. It covers it up. It stuffs down the flesh that needs to be exposed. It creates more problems in the process. When you eat to deal with difficult experiences, you aren't dealing with them. For example, you can set yourself up for anxiety and weight gain, because traumatic experiences then become unfinished business. Through eating, you learn to avoid dealing with the issues that cause you to eat.

Even if you stop eating and lose the weight, these issues will still be there. So, if you have a persistent weight problem, it is a good idea to consult a therapist to help you sort through the issues that caused you to gain weight and keep it on. It isn't easy to work through these problems, and sometimes it's downright painful, but in the long run, by confronting the demons that cause the behaviors you are likely to become more self-aware and better able to address behaviors and eliminate them as they occur. Fortunately, there are excellent types of therapy to help you deal with traumatic events, such as prolonged-exposure therapy for posttraumatic stress disorder. (In this treatment, clients learn to confront the memories of trauma and work through it. See the Notes and Resource sections for more information.)

SUBSTITUTING FOOD FOR LOVE

Do you ever crave food when you are actually craving love and support? Do you find that you eat when you want someone to hold you or nurture you? If so, you may substitute food for the love that you didn't receive as a child or to fill the lack of love in your life now.

There are two major problems in using food in this way. The first is that, because you substitute food, you make yourself less likely to find the love you crave. For instance, the more I used food to make up for the lack of support I found in my marriage, the more I felt that I didn't deserve the love I really wanted. I wanted to leave the marriage, but I feared that no one would love or want me. So I stayed—and I didn't get the caring treatment that I needed and deserved. In this way, food becomes the cure but also the cause.

The second problem is that you are likely to gain the weight back even if you lost it. Once the honeymoon with being thin ends, you may realize that you are still missing something critically valuable in your life: warm, loving relationships with a family member, spouse, or significant other.

FOOD NEVER JUDGES YOU

People who have experienced trauma, abuse, or the lack of validating relationships often seek validation. This means they want to find a way to feel good about themselves or at least to not feel so bad. When they become used to others who are critical, controlling, or judgmental, they look for ways to feel less negatively judged. Larina has heard people say, "Food is safe—it can't judge me." As weird as it may sound, it is hard to find something that makes you feel good that doesn't make you feel judged. Food provides instant positive reinforcement when you taste something that is enjoyable.

Ironically, trying to control your food often results in its controlling you. You eat and gain weight, and end up feeling more judged by others. When people try to control their uncontrollable lives through their eating, disorder eating habits typically result. Overeating, bulimia, and anorexia are all ways to attempt to control food, weight, or mood.

FOOD IS ALWAYS AVAILABLE

One of the main reasons that people who have endured difficult experiences turn to food is that it is there. Have you ever had the horrible experience of waking from a nightmare in the middle of the night and having no one there to soothe you? When you use food as your reassurance, you know that it is always available. It is hard to find something that is always there for you in the way that food is.

Food is also a socially acceptable way to deal with negative emotions and traumatic experiences. Many people who've been through trauma turn to drugs, alcohol, or abusive relationships as ways to cope. These methods are not socially acceptable in the way that food is. You could joke at work the next day about finishing your pint of double fudge brownie ice cream the night before, but a joke about finishing a bottle of vodka wouldn't be received the same way.

This is another reason that food feels like a "safe" mechanism for coping with life stress and pain. Again, there is an irony here, because food leads to weight gain and there is a negative view of obese people in society today. But in the moment, food can feel safe, or at least seem like the better choice. And often it is: it is difficult if not impossible to die of a french fry overdose, but you could overdose on heroin had you turned to drugs.

Nevertheless, when you get into a pattern of eating to stuff down your pain and hurt, that pain and hurt are likely to come out in other ways. If you have lost weight but not dealt with some of the hidden meanings that food has for you, then it's important to do so or you might just find that weight coming back.

TIP

Don't allow food to be your coping strategy. Make food less prevalent (don't keep bags of chips in your house!) and always keep positive coping strategies on hand. Write a list of positive coping strategies (walking, talking to a friend, writing in a journal, etc.) and be sure that at least three are always easy to access. If you rely on food to cover up traumatic memories or upsetting emotions, consider setting up a meeting with a professional to determine if psychotherapy can benefit you.

KEYS TO CHANGE

The first key to changing any hidden meanings of food is to realize exactly what food means to you. Even if you've been successful with weight loss, your real meaning of food can sabotage your weight loss. So the first question to ask yourself is how eating has related to the difficult experiences you've had. Think about some of the issues we've brought up in this chapter and some of the personal reasons that you have turned to food throughout your life.

If one of the main factors leading to your eating habits is the trauma you experienced, or if the traumatic event frequently comes up for you (in memories, nightmares, or flashbacks), or if you avoid thinking about the memory and things associated with the trauma, get a psychological evaluation to see if therapy can be helpful. Your experiences may need to be worked through and flushed out for you to feel better.

TIP

Don't underestimate the power of therapy or other forms of Thin Club member supports. Not getting help for past issues such as abuse, neglect, or other difficulties still affecting you can sabotage your Thin Club membership. See Chapter 8 for how to select a therapist.

Some types of therapy, such as prolonged-exposure therapy, which is a type of cognitive-behavioral therapy, are highly effective for processing trauma and overcoming the responses that drive you to eat. Prolonged-exposure therapy is a short-term therapy shown to be highly effective in dozens of research studies. For example, one study showed that people who had posttraumatic stress disorder significantly decreased anxiety and depression at the end of treatment. At a six-month follow-up, 75 percent of participants no longer had diagnosable posttraumatic stress. If you have symptoms, be sure to get proper treatment because it can greatly help you.

The second step is to work on the issues that drive you to eat. When you do this, food takes on a new meaning. It is no longer used to stuff down pain. Instead, it's used as a truly healthful way to provide your body with nutrients and energy. You then gain control and the food loses control over you.

The third step is to come up with alternative strategies to take the place of food. If food was replacing love or comfort for you, find other ways to receive love and comfort. For example, one of the best ways to find love is by giving it to others. Volunteer, mentor, take in a stray pet, or do other things that allow you to give love.

Desiree Ayres, a former Hollywood stuntwoman, battled eating disorders for much of her childhood and early adult life. Now the pastor at the In His Presence Church in the Warner Center, Woodland Hills, California, near Hollywood, Desiree relied on her spiritual connection to be healed of anorexia, bulimia, and compulsive binge eating. "I replaced food as a comfort source," she explains. "When you immerse yourself in the spiritual aspect of life, you don't have to fill yourself with food." Eventually, Desiree recognized a similar void in others, and people with weight issues began seeking her spiritual solace. She decided to share her inspirational story beyond her congregation and give her pointers for using religious principles to battle body issues. By helping others, she continued to keep herself on track.

Look for other ways to improve your life so food does not fill your voids. Practice living mindfully in the moment, not getting sucked into reliving your past. Of course, this does not mean you avoid thinking about your past, but you learn to fully experience the present. Even in difficult times, practice accepting the moment and not allowing it to damage your resolve to continue your healthy lifestyle.

TIP

Carpe diem. List ten ways you can work on seizing the day and living in the present moment. These can be as direct as noticing good things about the present moment or considering things you'd like to do with your time that you've been putting off or haven't yet accomplished. If, for example, you've always yearned to fly a plane, put it on your list and figure out how you can achieve it.

You can live mindfully in the moment by putting all of your attention into whatever you are currently doing. Allow yourself to experience the situation in a nonjudgmental and accepting manner. If you are going for a walk, simply go for a walk, without getting caught up in your concerns, worries, and inner turmoil. Take in the sights, smells, feelings of the air and the ground, and sounds of the animals or people around you. Focus on experiencing the world and keeping your attention on what is happening at that moment. Practice living mindfully in the moment during any of your daily activities.

FOUR

WHEN THE GOAL IS GONE

Creating New Goals to Keep You Inspired

WHEN I WAS 220+ POUNDS, MY GOAL WAS OBVI-
ous. I wanted to be thin. I didn't want to wear fat clothes
anymore. I wanted the inner me to burst through, and I
wanted the world to see who I really was. I wanted to stop
hiding behind my fat. I was bound and determined, and I
knew exactly what I wanted. I wanted to lose the weight!

Weight Watchers showed me my acceptable weight
range. And although it was far, far away and it seemed like
I'd never get anywhere near that goal, I knew exactly
where I was going. The cross-country trip had begun and I
was aiming for California—from New York, on foot! I was
determined to get there. California, here I come!

I took my weight-loss goals in small increments. Every
pound lost was a celebration! Ten pounds was even more
so. Could I make it to twenty? I challenged myself. And
while there were setbacks, plateaus, and such, I knew that
these were just rest stops on the highway. I didn't need a
GPS to know I was headed in the right direction.

The challenges became a game. Could I make it to 170?
Could I get below 150? Would I ever really be 130? When

something stalled, I pulled into a truck stop and tried to figure out what was going wrong. But then something strange happened. I got there. First, I was within my acceptable weight range. Then I was well within it. I had reached the goal. The scale was where I wanted it to be, and I was proud of my new dress size! But I was like a marathoner who finishes the long race. Although thrilled in one sense, I also faced an overwhelming sense of emptiness. I found myself facing the fact that my goal was gone. Now technically "thin" and presumably at goal, I faced a great big, "So, now what?" I had nothing left to work toward. A feeling of letdown took over. The letdown factor wasn't something I had anticipated when I tipped the scales at 225 pounds.

IT'S NOT ABOUT NUMBERS

Somewhere along the line I began to understand that, although I had physically achieved the goal, there was more to the goal than losing weight. Although the numbers were pretty much where I wanted them to be, there was more to setting a weight-loss goal than looking at numbers. Once I "achieved" the goal of fitting into the clothes I enjoy and getting the scale down to my comfort zone, I realized that the number on the scale and the label on the clothes are . . . well . . . just numbers. This is not to say that I ever want to see the scale go up, and I don't want to ever see myself in a larger dress size, but other goals are much more definitive and important.

The problem is that the numbers solve a problem, particularly for many of us who have been overweight and have an "internal barometer" problem. When we are heavy, we are not able to use just energy, mood, clothing, and mirrors to ascertain our weight and health. We have developed explanations and rationales, like "The cleaners shrunk my skirt" or "It was a diet muffin so I can have two"; they are ingrained in our pre- and post-weight-loss psyches. These barometers are hard to abandon when we reach our ideal weight, which is why we can't completely abandon the numbers on the scale or the clothing-size benchmarks when we reach our weight-loss goal. We have to use them judiciously to ascertain that we stay at goal.

I realized that I had a lot of work to do—and many more goals to address.

When I embarked on my journey, besides wanting to look great, I wanted to feel good, have more energy, and be healthy. I wanted to wear nice clothes and feel more comfortable in public. I wanted my outside appearance to match the personality that I always had on my inside. I wanted to find the courage to leave my unsatisfactory marriage and to find myself. I wanted to be a better and more energetic mother. I wanted to encourage my children to watch what they ate and enjoy exercise. And after some careful evaluation, I realized that, although the weight-loss goal may be gone, there were other challenges—in fact, many new goals—that I could set out to conquer.

I became more cognizant of my energy level, moods, feelings, and certainly of my health as I became thinner. I began to work on my comfort level in public. My children joined me in exercising and eating right, becoming healthier along with me. I used my higher energy level to play tennis with them and take them kickboxing. And, of course, one of my new goals became writing this book to help others deal with their post-weight-loss issues. And that, for me, has been one more step en route to not just one but a whole host of new goals.

THE MOTIVATION

Having a very specific and measurable weight-loss goal is a huge motivator. Clear, concise goals are one of the most accurate predictors of whether or not people can achieve a major behavioral change. If you were successful with your weight loss, you likely had a clear goal in mind that you pursued until you achieved it. You channeled your energy into turning your dream into reality and recognized your progress along the way. You delighted in those times that you could push the scale down a notch or tighten your belt. There are many great rewards along the way of losing weight, and these little rewards keep you focused on achieving your goal.

But now what? You've achieved the goal, so why do you need to continue pursuing it? That doesn't make any sense and you can be left in a state of confusion. You may lose the motivation to continue making healthful eating choices and exercising regularly. It's much more difficult to stay motivated because you lose the exciting reward of weight loss. In the process of losing weight, you got the rush of seeing the scale drop down a pound or two, but you don't get the same rush seeing it stay the same. So, after you've achieved your goal, your focus must change and the work that you need to do also changes.

Top researchers in the treatment of obesity at Oxford University are now breaking weight-loss treatments into two distinct entities: the *weight-loss phase* and the *maintenance phase.* Many people completely neglect the maintenance phase. They think that they've reached the finish line and they're done. This is why most people gain the weight back. It's like buying a beautiful new home and then doing nothing to keep it up—it won't be beautiful and problem free for long!

The maintenance phase is important and requires some ongoing work and dedication. The way to think about it is: It's not that you now have *no* goal, it's that you have a *different* goal.

TIP

Create your moving target. When you come up with goals for yourself, think of them in succession or as a series of several goals. This will keep you moving forward and will help you continue to strive to make additional accomplishments now that you've met your weight-loss goal.

Your earlier goal was to enter The Thin Club. Now you're in it and your goal changes. Beware: If you have no goal and your plan is to coast along, you're likely to drift right back to where you were—out the door of the club. So let's create some new objectives.

GOING AFTER NEW GOALS

If you haven't already done this for yourself, now is the time to create some powerful new goals. The good news is that you can create targets that will help you keep the weight off and improve your life and health. These new targets can be goals related to the quality of the food you eat, an athletic or fitness goal, maintaining your weight loss, or improving other parts of yourself, now that you are happier with your body. Here are some examples of new goals that you can pursue.

Goals:

- Improve your fat-to-muscle ratio.
- Eat at least seven servings of fruits and vegetables per day.
- Create a new wardrobe style for your new body.
- Focus on advancing your career to the next level.
- Enhance the communications in your relationship.
- Find a new relationship.
- Eat more organic foods.
- Continue to lose weight at the slow rate of one to two pounds per month for the next year.
- Adopt a new sport or activity that you never thought you could handle before.
- Train for and run a marathon.
- Increase the weight that you can lift.
- Spend more time with family members.
- Create muscle definition where you never saw it before.

As you can see from this list, there are *tons* of new aspirations that you can create for yourself. The key is to pick a couple of objectives that motivate *you*. Select at least one that relates to maintaining or furthering your weight loss. Then add some that address other areas in your life. When you are happier and more fulfilled in general, you will be better equipped to keep your weight off.

Once you select some goals, increase the likelihood that you will achieve them by putting them into SMART goals. The concept of SMART goals was created by an unknown marketing and motivational genius. *SMART* stands for: *S*pecific, *M*easurable, *A*ction-oriented, *R*ealistic, and *T*imed. When you put your goals into this format, you increase the odds that you'll reach them. When new clients come to Larina and say the weight-loss goals they've been working on, she can predict whether they have achieved them based on the way they say the goals. Hint: When the goal is expressed in the SMART format, it's much more likely that it can be achieved.

For example, instead of saying, "Increase the weight that I can lift," which is vague and too broad to be a SMART goal, say, "Increase the weight I can lift for bicep curls from five pounds each to ten pounds each for three sets of twelve by the beginning of April." See how this intention is more motivating? It's measurable and specific—you'll know when you achieve it!

TIP

Write down your SMART goals. The best way to accomplish your goals is to express them in the SMART format. Then review them on a regular basis to see how you're progressing.

IF I'M NOT FAT, WHO AM I?

Along with uncertain goals can come a strange identity crisis. For example, I was always fat, so I knew how to relate to the world as a fat person. But forging a new identity—that was baffling to me. Trying on new identities has become like trying on shoes. Some fit, and some pinch and don't quite fit comfortably. But, ah, the shopping trip can be one delightful experience! Hence, you may want to create some goals to help you find your new identity.

Many people have developed an identity that goes along with their weight. This is particularly true for those who have been overweight for much of their lives. Identity development is intense during adolescence. If you were overweight or obese as a teenager, some part of your identity is likely to be wrapped up in being a heavy person.

But when you lose a substantial amount of weight, you become a different person in many ways. You feel different. You look different. People treat you differently. In reality, a good portion of your identity is called into question. This can be troubling for some people because they feel that they don't know what their new identity is.

For example, someone who was on a tour with Larina during a whitewater rafting vacation consistently made fat jokes about himself. The operator had to balance the weights in the raft, and he joked that he'd take one side and the other seven people could take the other side to balance him out. He was very funny and kept the group laughing, but of course it made Larina realize how much this participant's identity was wrapped up in being the "fat funny person." If he loses the weight, what will he joke about? Would he still be funny? Are his jokes, which are designed to protect him, actually hurting him? Self-deprecating humor usually deprecates the self.

Jessica Fischer, a woman who was on *The Jane Pauley Show* with us, had been a comedienne before she lost half her body weight via gastric bypass surgery. After she lost the weight, she didn't feel funny anymore. She wasn't sure that a skinny person telling the same jokes would be found funny by the audience; she was left with a lack of identity and faced the monumental task of forging a new identity. Her struggle with this process of identity change is shown in an award-winning documentary, *What's So Funny?*

You may encounter a struggle with identity following your weight loss. Here are some exercises that Larina recommends; try them out to see what happens.

To find yourself:

- First, create a list of your core values. These are the things that matter most to you and that you could not live your life without.
- Next, create a list of how you believe others saw you before the weight loss. Now do the same thing for how people view you following your weight loss.
- Make a list of how you view yourself pre- and post-weight-loss. Try to focus on positive qualities that make up the essence of who you are, rather than appearance-oriented qualities.

See what is consistent in the pre and post lists for how you view yourself and how others view you: This is the identity you currently have. There are likely to be parts that you like and parts you'd like to change. Compare these qualities with your core values. When an aspect of yourself doesn't match up with your core values, that is an identity problem that you may want to address. To do this, begin by acting in a manner more consistent with the qualities that you desire and value. Try it on for size, just as you try on new sizes of clothes. It may feel awkward at first, but if you practice living the way you want to live, your sense of your identity will follow suit.

LABELS AND LANGUAGE

The language and the labels that we use with ourselves are part of our identity. For instance, we have a way to talk with ourselves. This language does not necessarily change when you lose weight. For instance, if you used to think "I'm fat; I should not wear clothes like that" or "I should not let people see me eating since I am so heavy," you are likely to retain these thoughts after the weight loss. This leads to confusion, negative emotions, and questioning: "Who am I now that I am thin?" So, the next step in creating a new identity for yourself is to change your self-talk and your labels. In the last step, Larina recommended bringing your behaviors in line with your desired new identity. When you combine these new actions with new thoughts, you will find a synergistic effect.

Begin by becoming aware of what you say to yourself. Recognize *what* you say and *when* you say it. Write these things down. For example, you may catch yourself saying, "I just sat on the couch for an hour, I'm so lazy!" Now ask yourself whether these thoughts are consistent with your new behavior and your desired identity. If you are now an active person who exercises several times a week, you are not lazy.

So the next step is to change the labels. Write down an alternative way of responding to the situation. You could say, "I just sat down for an hour because I'm exhausted after a long day and I needed to relax. I had a great workout this morning and I'm not lazy."

Remember: Many people will treat you as the "old" you, even though you've made some changes in your identity. For now, just focus on how you can change what you do and how you talk with yourself. This will help you create the identity and self-esteem that you want and deserve.

TIP

Be aware of the labels and language you use with yourself. Describe yourself in terms of the *state* rather than the *trait*. That is, rather than assign global and stable characteristics, focus on the current situation—what's going on around you and your state of mind. This process will also help you set realistic goals because you'll see that aspects of yourself and your motivation wax and wane with time. If you are ravenous one day after a heavy workout, you may in fact need some additional calories. This does not make you a "pig" or a "failure" at weight maintenance.

CUT THE CRITICISM

Building a Better Body Image

No, you are not my type at all. I don't go for heavy women, and even though I was being nice on our date, you still look it! The same attitude that precluded you from going to my house on a first date (believe me, I wasn't about to jump on you, Fat Girl) is exactly what separates us, and why meeting you was a total waste of my time (and many, many women have trusted me enough to come here for a first date, because there is no reason not to trust me, I am a lawyer, for goodness sake).

The e-mail from *Mr. Attorney* was waiting in my in-box shortly after I returned from our disappointingly dismal date. We had met in person for a quick drink in a noisy bar. He was an ugly man with a splintery gray beard, ruddy complexion, stooped posture, and droopy blue jeans. Although he claimed to be my age, he looked about ten years older than me and his eyes watered during the conversation as if he were about to burst into tears.

I was polite but distant, trying to remain cheerful during the date. He was clearly depressed, and after about a half hour of talking about what each of us was looking for in a new mate, he sprung up from the table and said, "I want to leave now." I didn't want to date him again. In fact, I was hugely relieved when we left the bar. And I was happy that I had had enough self-respect and regard for my safety and welfare to decline his initial invitation to meet at his house. In my former state of low self-esteem, I might have succumbed.

His e-mail calling me "heavy" might have devastated the fat girl who used to dwell within me, possibly sending me back to the pastries. I might have thrown away the pantsuit I had worn, positive that it wasn't flattering and that I really did look fat. But something had changed. Me! The Me who used to change my clothes fifteen times before I left the house because whatever I was wearing made me look "too fat!" The Me who used to check every mirror I walked by to see which part of me was bulging, hanging, or looking less than perfect. The Me who, after my weight loss, so desperately craved approval that I wouldn't leave the house without flawless makeup and perfect clothing. And as I deleted his nasty e-mail, it suddenly occurred to me that I no longer needed a man to tell me I was thin and beautiful. This man's electronic missile had missed its mark entirely.

Instead of taking his criticism to heart, feeling sad or wondering how much of what he said was true, this new member of The Thin Club looked in the mirror, saw my new toned body, and felt proud! I flexed my muscles once or twice for good measure. Oh, yes, that pantsuit definitely was flattering. I knew who I was. Body image is intact and, in fact, doing fine.

WHAT'S A BODY IMAGE?

We're sure you're familiar with the term "body image." You may have heard people say things like "He has a negative body image" or "She has a healthy body image." But what does this really mean? In this chapter, we'll talk about your body image before and after your weight loss, and the issues you will face as your body (and your body image) changes.

Your body image is your relationship with your body. Like a relationship with someone else, there are several components, including the physical aspect, your own unique perceptions, and the emotional aspect of that association.

THE PHYSICAL ASPECT

As the name implies, your body image has to do with the image you have of your body. It includes what you see when you look in the mirror. Some of what you see is based on the objective physical reality of your appearance; these are the things that others see as well. If you have hair down to your waist, you see long hair. If you have a bald head, you see a bald head.

People, especially women, learn to internalize both the things they hear about their own bodies and the things they hear others say about their bodies (for example, if a girl grows up hearing her mom complain about her thighs, she'll start to worry about her own thighs). People are also influenced by the standards of beauty in their culture, which is why body image in some cultures is much more accepting and positive than in others. When you have a healthy body image, the negative comments of others roll off, but hearing positive things from others can help you develop a healthy body image.

We are typically our own worst enemy when it comes to body image (we see all the problem areas that others may not notice), but people who have heard negative comments from others are even worse enemies to themselves. Fortunately, when people lose weight they receive a lot of favorable comments from people, which can help them shift their own body images and gain confidence.

TIP

Listen to the favorable comments you hear as you lose weight and use them as a body-image booster shot.

A friend of mine recently lost about forty pounds. While she has another forty pounds to go, she is rightfully proud of her shrinking body—proud enough to pull out a twenty-five-year-old photo of herself and show it to people, asking, "Do I look the same as I did then?"

I was appalled when a mutual friend shook her head and said, "Of course, you don't look like that—you were twenty-eight years old in that photo, for goodness sake!" Naturally, the woman administering the comment has her own body-image issues. She has been trying unsuccessfully to lose weight for years. If you have heard negative comments about your body, Larina encourages you to think of the people who said them and realize why those people said them. The comments are usually more about the person who said them and the individual's own insecurities and issues than about you. Ask yourself: What is she rejecting or criticizing about herself? But don't spend too long psychoanalyzing her. Some people just aren't worth the time, and they have the negative ability to pull you down into the lake along with them. It is better to focus on yourself—your own success and your own goals. As you become more confident in your abilities and your body image, you will bounce back from these remarks a lot faster.

TIP

Do you still feel fat even though you're not? Decide what size you think you still are or look like. Let's say you decide on size 16. Then go into a store and try on clothes of this size. How do they look? Chances are, they are too big! Then try on something the size you really are to show yourself the difference.

YOUR OWN PERCEPTION OF YOURSELF

Sometimes a change in a physical aspect of your body can enhance your body image. This is like an attraction to your mate. If you are attracted to him as he is, but he makes a nice change in the way he dresses and does his hair, your attraction may increase somewhat. While physical attributes affect your body image, much of it also is about your own perception. For this reason, neither an extreme makeover, a significant weight loss, or a radical surgical intervention is likely to completely transform your body image. Larina frequently hears from clients who have lost a lot of weight that they still see their former selves in the mirror despite the dramatic changes that have occurred.

Some people look in the mirror and see something distorted, like in a fun house. This distortion can occur no matter what your weight. For example, anorexic patients who weigh seventy-five pounds are at one extreme end of having a distorted body image. They look in the mirror and see fat where other people see just skin and bones. This distortion of their body image is clearly unhealthy. People die from anorexia nervosa because they believe they are chubby; they so intensely fear becoming fat that they won't allow themselves to eat so much as a cracker.

At the other end are obese people who see themselves as physically fit and healthy. This body-image distortion can also be unhealthy. For instance, when I was heavy, I looked in the mirror and told myself I was muscular. The muscles were, unfortunately, buried under a whole lot of fat. "Big boned" is another euphemism some people use to describe their heavy bodies. While we are huge advocates of body acceptance, we do not promote body *denial*. There is a wealth of scientific data showing that people who are clinically or morbidly obese are more susceptible to dozens of health problems, one of which is increased mortality, which means they're more likely to *die*. Thinking that you are fit and healthy despite 100 extra pounds on your body is denial.

THE EMOTIONAL ASPECT

The other aspect of body image is your emotions. Think of the last time you got into an argument with your spouse or significant other. Once you got all worked up and angry, did you begin to see everything that he or she did as annoying and irritating? Emotions can cloud our thought processes and judgment in all aspects of life, including body image. If you feel down, blue, or fatigued, you may look at yourself more negatively than when you feel cheerful and energetic.

TIP

What's your body image now? Look in the mirror for one minute and observe yourself. Then, right down the first twenty words that come into your mind about how you appear. Try not to put thought into it; just jot down what pops into your head. These words will give you an idea of your body image. If your list is clouded with more negative words than positive ones, you may want to find a way to address your body-image issues, either through therapy or by using some of the techniques described here.

For many of us, body image is created during adolescence. In a study, those who were overweight or obese as teens showed higher body-image dissatisfaction even after weight loss. Their body image had solidified during their teens and stuck around even after the weight came off. On the other hand, those who became obese later in life had body-image satisfaction following weight loss similar to people of normal weight who had no history of obesity.

BODY IMAGE ISN'T MEASURED IN POUNDS OR KILOGRAMS

You may assume that everyone who loses weight automatically gains a positive body image. This isn't true! And it is disappointing for those who expect to suddenly have a positive body image after weight loss to discover that they still don't have one.

While studies show that body image typically improves with weight loss, larger weight losses are not associated with greater improvements in body image. Instead, it is hypothesized that smaller weight losses lead to improved body image. However, further improvements don't occur with more weight loss. This shows that there is no direct relationship between body image and weight or weight loss.

You may have noticed that body image and weight aren't always related. Say you know a thin friend who obsesses about the cellulite on her thighs and does not have a healthy body image. You yourself may still have concerns about round cheeks despite your weight loss. You might know other people who are several pounds overweight who are the life of the party, who get all the nice-looking guys, and who are happy overall with who they are and how they interact with others.

Some studies have shown that body image improves equally when people receive cognitive-behavioral therapy and don't lose weight as when people don't receive therapy but do lose weight. That is, changing your thinking and behavior can lead to a better body image even if you don't lose weight.

TIP

Do you find yourself comparing your body to others? Write down all the thoughts that come into your mind about someone else's physique. Then write down all the thoughts about your own. Compare the two lists. Then look at the lists objectively to see how true the thoughts really are. You may need to get some assistance from an objective observer to compare the lists.

There is also research that suggests a negative body image can persist even after weight has come off. In one study, normal-weight women who had lost significant weight had high body-image dissatisfaction. They also had high discrepancies between their ideal weight and their current weight and increased anxiety about being weighed. The weight may go away, but the body-image problems can stick around. So how do we begin to eliminate the negative, as the song says?

Some of The Thin Club members I spoke to used hypnotherapy and exercise to help them focus on positive aspects of their bodies. Others found therapy or support groups a helpful solution. Still others I've interviewed used prayer and turned toward a higher power to help them recognize that their body was made in God's image and therefore is perfect. I used a combination of these solutions to help me celebrate my new body. Belly dancing, for example, is one of the most in-your-face forms of exercise a person could choose to enjoy. I added it to my exercise routine, enjoying the sheer cardiovascular benefits and the arm work, and the movement of my not-too-flat mommy tummy—after all, what good is belly dancing with no belly at all? By the end of my first round of classes, I was ready to bare more than I ever thought I'd dare.

TIP

What was your teenage body image? Since a good deal of your body image is formed during your teenage years, reminding yourself of your teen body image can give you insights into not only how you feel about your looks but also how you respond to weight-related situations today. Write down all the words that describe how you felt about and saw your body as a teenager. Then compare this list with the one you created from looking in the mirror now. Has it changed? Is it the same? If the change is for the positive, chart your growth. If it has remained the same, note where you need encouragement and improvement. Then choose a method of addressing your weaker areas. Simple solutions may exist. For instance, a girl who felt flat-chested as a teen may have developed into a woman who is embarrassed about her breast size or shape. She could solve the problem at the nearest Victoria's Secret, buying the sexiest push-up bra in the store.

ACCEPTANCE

While certain things will change when you lose weight, others may remain the same. For example, you may always have a round belly. Your legs may always rub together when you walk. Love handles may never be completely absent from your life. You may always have some underarm fat that flaps when you wave good-bye. Even after you have lost the weight, you will have to accept that all the dieting in the world won't change what nature has bestowed upon you. Age, skin elasticity, hormones, and genetics are life's basic "givens" and they will not change radically just because you have slimmed down.

Because of this, one of the first steps to a positive body image is acceptance. The more you get frustrated by and resist your body's natural tendencies, the more you will feel dissatisfied and upset. Research shows that a good deal of what determines body type is inherited. This means that your appearance, like your height, is in your genes and there isn't much you can do about it.

For instance, some people are built as pears and others as apples. Some are muscular and bulky, others are petite. Observing people of different ethnicities and races will show you the biological components of body types. Some are tall and thin and others are naturally voluptuous. Of course, you can modify the shape of your body through diet and exercise, but there is a point where you must accept that you are what you are.

Body acceptance is an important element of successful weight loss, no matter where you are in the process. Whether you are still working on losing weight or you are already a member of The Thin Club, a key to meeting your goals is accepting your current body.

So how do you accept your body? Keep in mind that acceptance is different from love. If you still have fifty pounds to lose and don't love how you look right now, that's OK—but you can accept it. Acceptance is a nonjudgmental quality. It means that you pass no judgment on yourself regarding your appearance.

TIP

Try to catch yourself whenever you make a critical comment to yourself about your appearance or weight. Then replace the judgmental thought with a neutral description. Go from "I hate the way my tummy protrudes in this dress" to "I've tried on more flattering clothes. It's amazing the way certain styles can make you look larger." If you avoid making negative statements to yourself and still do not have a favorable body image, work on saying more positive statements to yourself. For example, give yourself a compliment for an aspect of your appearance that looks nice.

WHAT'S NICE ABOUT ME?

Even in our largest and most cumbersome stages, there is usually something nice we can find about our bodies. Eyes are seldom fat—and often very beautiful. Hands can be delicate and fingers tapered, even in the throes of a weight loss. Learn to recognize, celebrate, and adorn your nicest features, even when you're feeling self-conscious about your body. Make a list of your best features and post it somewhere visible.

Another way to accept your body is to get accustomed to it. Those who are overweight often report avoiding looking at themselves. Even with no one else present in the room, they often get dressed and undressed in the dark and avoid looking in the mirror. To help desensitize yourself to views of your own body, stop these avoidances. If it feels too difficult to look at yourself undressed in the mirror, look at yourself partially dressed or keep the lights dimmed. Work your way up to the most frightening situation, which is usually looking at yourself nude in broad daylight. The key to making this desensitization exercise successful is practicing use of nonjudgmental language with yourself. If you find yourself saying, "Augh, look at that roll of fat!" end the experience and begin it again a minute later. Continue to repeat it until you can do it without making negative judgments.

CHANGING YOUR BELIEFS

Do you hold assumptions about how you look and come across to others? You might not know whether you do or not, so be on the lookout for them. A great way to spot an assumption is to look for the words *should* or *must*. Here are some examples.

Assumptions:

- I must be in shape to be worthwhile.
- I should always present my best appearance when in public.
- My appearance should show who I am inside (you are what you eat).

Another common assumption is that you cannot like yourself without liking your appearance. Or that others will not like you if you don't look a certain way. Or that you cannot feel good about yourself with all the images of skinny models in the media. The best way to tackle these assumptions is to realize that they are assumptions. They are based on the word *assume.* You don't know these things for a fact. They feel true because you have heard them for a long time and have come to believe them. Instead of accepting these ideas as undeniable truths, find out just how true they really are.

Question them. Compare them to your core values to see how they measure up. If you say, "I must be in shape to be worthwhile," that implies that only thin people are worthwhile. Do you really believe that? What qualities are more important to you than being thin? What about being a good-hearted person? What about being generous and kind? How about your intelligence and ambition? These all sound like worthwhile qualities.

If you hold the assumption that you cannot like yourself without liking your appearance, then you may be at risk of losing your Thin Club membership. If you only like yourself because you are thin, what happens if you have a "fat day," or you get pregnant, or you gain a few pounds back? Holding on to this assumption is like holding on to a box of crème-filled donuts—risky! Overcome this assumption by focusing on liking other parts of yourself. These may be other aspects of your appearance or things com-pletely unrelated to your body.

If you believe that others will not like you if you don't look a certain way, ask yourself how true this idea is. Cer-tainly there is some appearance and weight discrimination out there, but is it really true that *most* people won't like you if you do not look a certain way? And if it were true that someone didn't like you because of your appearance, would that be someone you'd even want to like you or be friends with? It's important to question these assumptions even if you are now thin; you don't want to put undue pressure on yourself, which will make you more likely to become heavy again.

What about the belief that you cannot feel good about yourself with all those images of skinny models in the media? Larina hears this from people even after they've lost substantial weight and have gone down several sizes. At first these women said they wanted to weigh 160. Then it became 150. When they reached 140, they were not happy because they compared themselves to size 2 models or size 4 friends and they still felt big. The best way to overcome this belief is to purposefully adopt a new, more healthy and positive one.

TIP

Change your idea of "perfect." Decide right now that you will not use the 0.5 percent of the population with "perfect" bodies as a yardstick for how you should look. Focus on your success and the strength that it took to get there. Realize that there's much more to leading a great life than having the "perfect" body and that no one has the perfect life, even those who look perfect.

BEHAVIORS FOR A BETTER BODY IMAGE

You have changed your eating behaviors, but if you keep doing negative things, you might be unable to change your view of your body. This is because certain behaviors are likely to keep a negative body image around, even after you've lost weight. These negative behaviors fall into two types: *avoidance* and *rituals*. For example, people who are overweight get into the habit of avoiding certain situations. Some of the common situations are weighing yourself, going to doctors, being photographed or videotaped, wearing certain types of clothing like bathing suits or tight-fitting clothes, sexual activity, shopping, approaching attractive people in social situations, striking certain poses, and looking in the mirror. Do you avoid any of these things?

Ritualistic behaviors include checking and fixing aspects of your appearance. You may check your weight frequently by getting on the scale a couple of times every day. You check over and over how you look in certain outfits. You look in the mirror and think, "Does my butt look too big in these jeans?" You walk away and return again for another look. Checking can also involve asking others for reassurance. You could ask this question of someone else ("Does my butt look too big in these jeans?"), hoping for an answer that will calm your fears. "Fixing" rituals are done throughout the day. You fix your shirt to hide your stomach. You fix your hair or your makeup whenever you go to the restroom. You change your clothes and then change again and again before deciding what to wear when you go out. Do you have any rituals like these?

These avoidance and ritualistic behaviors increase

anxiety, distress, and self-consciousness. The solution is surprisingly simple: Do the things you avoid and don't do the rituals. Believe it or not, you can *act* your way to a healthy body image. That is, when you learn that you can experience those things that you've been avoiding and feel OK, you become more comfortable and confident.

If the situations that you normally avoid are too intimidating to face up front, break them up into smaller chunks. If wearing a swimming suit at a public pool feels unbearable, for instance, begin by wearing shorts and a T-shirt. Your next step may be a sleeveless shirt or shorter pair of shorts. Then you go to the pool and keep your T-shirt on. Next, you wear your swimming suit in the lounge chair without getting up. Finally, you wear your swimming suit to the pool and walk around and swim.

The great thing about ending your avoidances is that you kill two birds with one stone: You become less self-conscious and uncomfortable and you experience enjoyable activities that before you'd avoided. In the past, you sat around sweating on a ninety-degree day, and now you can cool off in a nice pool and relax in the sun.

Likewise, the best way to stop ritualistic behaviors is to end them cold turkey. Just don't do them. Try not to check yourself and your outfits. Weigh yourself only once per day. Don't ask someone if your butt looks big. (The answer never makes you feel better anyway, right?) If you have difficulty stopping cold turkey, begin by delaying the rituals. Tell yourself that you will wait for an hour before looking in the mirror. Postpone changing your outfit until after you wore the current outfit for thirty minutes. What you are doing is gaining control of your urges and not letting them control you. Over time these urges will decrease and your confidence will increase.

Another option is to put limits on your ritualistic behaviors. Tell yourself that you have only fifteen minutes to get dressed, so you can't try on every outfit in your closet. Say that you will purchase at least one item of clothing while shopping to resist the urge to search for the "perfect" outfit that disguises all your perceived flaws.

When you change your thought processes, assumptions, and behaviors in the way that we've described here, you will slowly notice changes in your body image. You will begin by accepting yourself. You will grow to have a positive relationship with your body, with a healthy body image and a greater sense of self-assurance. These changes will make you less susceptible to difficulties that occur with weight loss and maintenance. A healthy body image is an insurance policy for your membership in The Thin Club.

TIP

Sunday exhibitionist. This works best in the summer or when you are on vacation. Choose your skimpiest outfit or bathing suit and wear it all day with no butt-hiding jacket or beach cover-up. Flaunt your body for all to see. Practice a sexy walk to augment the new you. Stifle all impulses to hide or mask body parts. Work it! After all, you are a member of The Thin Club now!

SIX

RISKY TIMES

Dealing with Backslide Temptations

I HATE MOVING. I'VE DONE IT SEVERAL TIMES IN THE past few years and somehow it never gets any easier. About one-third of the way down to my goal weight, while I was still married, my family moved to a new town. After unpacking loads of boxes, learning about the school district, exploring the shopping venues, joining the local synagogue, and introducing myself to the neighbors, I felt the need to turn my house into a home. I proceeded to do what I know how to do best. I cooked and I baked.

I baked cookies, cakes, and pies (allowing myself just a bite of this and a smidge of that and licking the batter—'cause batter licking doesn't count a bit when you're on a diet!). And sugar being the addictive substance that it is, one bite was never enough. By cooking and baking, I felt that I was somehow marking my territory, filling the house with good vibes and smells and dealing with the stress of being in a new town and having to make new friends. Eventually, I had to buy a second refrigerator/freezer to store all the home-baked treats. I began sending out the extras as care packages to soldiers in Iraq. Then the dinner invitations from friendly neighbors began to flow, and as the neighborhood began to chatter and buzz about the homemade desserts I would bring with me to their elegant dinner parties, my waistline slowly began to expand. My neighborliness was putting me back in the fat zone!

But I realized somewhere along the line, through hypnosis and introspection, that my backslide had nothing to do with being a good neighbor. In analyzing the *why* of my lack of self-control, I realized that the move had left me feeling stressed out, disconnected, lonely, and somewhat depressed. The baking, while it was my way of turning my house into a home, with the wafting odor of cinnamon-nut mandlebread greeting people as they stopped in to say hello, was also my way of anesthetizing my mind from the trauma of a difficult change. Although I welcomed the move, welcomed the new friends and neighbors, I was facing the fears that many people face with a new move: Will I fit in? Will people like me? Will I find friends? And as I baked my way into other people's hearts, I threatened to destroy my heart in the process!

STRESS!

Looking back at my life, I realized that stressors have played a major role in my backslides whenever I had lost weight. My difficult marriage, coping with new children, dealing with a child's illness, the moves, and, most of all, coping with social pressures had caused me to regain weight even when I was looking my best.

The backslide might start with a small and innocuous piece of ice cream cake at a birthday party, usually on a day when I was feeling particularly stressed out and hungry because I had skipped lunch. Or it might begin with something that I'm "allowed," like a sugar-free pastry, that escalates into several pastries, and is followed by a sugar-free turnover to top it off. Or it might be portion sizes that exceed what I know I should have (instead of a handful of nuts, a bowlful, or two chicken breasts instead of one). And like the old Alka-Seltzer commercial, "I can't believe I ate the *whole thing!*" is the unfortunate end result. Like everything else associated with weight loss, it's about toning your mind!

PREVENTING THE BACKSLIDE

Even though we are living, breathing testaments for conquering temptation, there will be times—some more universal than others—when we are tempted to backslide. Like the Halloween candy bag that glows in the dark with your favorite candy, or the ungodly boyfriend whose breakup sends you running to the nearest bag of taco chips, these are challenges that on some level we've mastered, but on another we must always prepare for.

There are three major danger zones to look out for when you've lost weight. These are the warning signs that you may begin to put the weight back on, either gradually or quickly. The first is when you've caved in and eaten three pieces of cheesecake or five slices of pizza. You've "messed up" and are getting nervous about a backslide. The second is when negative emotions strike, and the third is a very common excuse that we bet you've said to yourself. When you know these potential danger zones and some strategies for managing them, you'll be able to handle the risky time with ease.

SOMEBODY SAVE ME! WHEN YOU CAVE IN

Just when you are finally used to living thin, something happens—perhaps a setback at home or at work—and you find yourself slipping into your old eating habits, which of course results in a weight gain. How do you keep yourself from backsliding completely? Is there a surefire way to put on the brakes when you find yourself starting to slip?

Fortunately, yes, there is. What Larina is about to share with you is perhaps the single most important point in making sure that you don't regain the weight. Ready? Read this carefully: It does not matter if you slip up and overeat one day. Everybody does this, even those people who have been thin their whole lives. *What matters is how you interpret the backslide.*

While it is certainly not ideal that you gave in to a moment of weakness and devoured six peanut butter cups, those six peanut butter cups will not make you regain all of your weight. You are absolutely right that you *can* start down a slippery slope. What starts you on the slippery slope is the way you interpret having eaten all that chocolate and peanut butter. Here are the interpretations most likely to result in a backslide:

1. "I've ruined my diet and now I'm back to square one."
2. "Now that I've failed, I might as well keep eating."
3. "See, I knew I was weak and have no willpower."
4. "Everyone said I couldn't do it and they were right."
5. "Life is so much better/easier/more enjoyable with lots of peanut butter cups, I might as well give up trying to be healthy."

As you can see, each of these interpretations puts the food or other people in control. These beliefs render you powerless and drain your motivation. The conclusions are also inaccurate. There is no way you gained back all of the weight you lost with one slip-up. Even if your slip-up was a major binge in which you consumed 3,500 calories, you'd gain back only one pound. We imagine that you lost more than one pound, so you certainly did not go back to square one.

The slippery slope is there because you let it be there. These conclusions are disguised excuses that enable you to keep eating. If you responded differently, you'd stop the backslide immediately. For example, you could say to yourself, "The peanut butter cups were not the healthiest selection, so I'm going to commit to a healthy dinner this evening and get myself right back on track. If I crave a peanut butter cup in the future, I will have a miniature one."

Personal trainer and nutritionist Steve Olschwanger has an awesome analogy. He likens those who cave on a backslide to those who trash their automobile after getting a flat tire. "When you get a flat tire, you fix it or replace the tire and keep on going," he says. "When you backslide on your diet, the same attitude applies."

TIP

Tone your mind by heightening your awareness of how you interpret a backslide. The first step is always to observe how you tend to handle setbacks. Be aware of your responses so you can change them. The second step is to handle them differently. If you notice an interpretation that looks like one of the five above, write it down. Then think of another way of responding that will be less likely to result in a backslide.

NEGATIVE EMOTIONS:
THE STRESS-FAT CONNECTION

It's important to improve how you handle negative moods because those negative moods can cause you to gain weight. There are two reasons for this. First, your appetite or food cravings may increase and you may eat more fattening foods. Second, your body may actually physically respond to the stress.

Findings from a research study at the Rush University Medical Center in Chicago showed that significant levels of stress led to increased conservation of fat. This may be because stress impacts the hormones involved with eating and metabolism. In addition, when you are chronically stressed your energy is lower and you are more likely to eat sugary foods to gain energy. You are also less likely to get yourself to the gym because you feel overwhelmed and exhausted by the stress.

TIP

Beat stress by managing your time and giving yourself at least 60 minutes a day of downtime or enjoyable activities. Even though it may feel as though you don't have time for such a luxury, relaxation time will help you beat stress and stay in The Thin Club!

Breaking the Food-Mood Association

How many times have you run for the cheesiest, greasiest, sweetest, most decadent, or chocolaty food you could find when you felt stressed or depressed? We all have! Negative emotions are tightly linked with making poor food choices, binge eating, and eating for comfort rather than to satisfy hunger or for nutrition. If you have lost a good amount of weight but still do not have your emotional eating under control, the weight loss may not last.

Most people who are "emotional eaters" know that they are. Are you? What emotions trigger cravings for you? Emotional eating is more than responding to cravings. It is when you eat a particular food in response to a feeling. It is also eating as a way of dealing with an emotion. As you probably know, eating is not the best way to cope with negative feelings.

Emotional eating puts you at risk of backsliding because inevitably you will experience the emotion that triggers your overeating. We will never have lives free of negative emotions that surface from time to time. If you haven't learned how to break the association between these feelings and certain foods, you will be at risk to regain weight.

The first step in breaking the cycle of emotional eating is to recognize your patterns. Larina recommends that you keep a log of the situation, the emotion, the food eaten, and the emotion after you ate the food. This will help you to see several things. First, you'll spot the mood that leads to binge eating. Second, you'll see which feelings are linked with which foods. You may find that you crave salty snacks when you're stressed, chocolate when you're depressed, and so on. Third, you'll see that the foods rarely relieve the feelings. In fact, they often intensify them.

Once you know the patterns, you can break them. The best way to break a bad habit is by making it impossible to do. If you know you crave caramel corn when you're angry, next time you're angry, keep away from any place that you could get caramel corn. The more times you are angry and don't have caramel corn, the sooner you'll break the connection. Your mind will form a new pattern in which caramel corn is not connected to the anger. For this reason, it's important that you experience that emotion many times without reaching for the food you crave so you can break the association.

TIP

Know which emotions trigger cravings for particular foods and then steer clear of those foods when you have that emotion. Remember that each time you have the emotion without having the food you'll weaken the association. Give yourself credit for each time you're able to have the emotion without caving in to the craving.

Another important strategy is to learn how to handle the emotions themselves. If you find that a particular feeling, like anxiety, is common for you, work on managing that anxiety. For example, you may choose to enroll in psychotherapy. Alternatively, you can begin a self-help program and read about constructive ways to handle the destructive behaviors that frequently accompany negative emotions. It is very important to learn how to handle the emotion because you don't want to substitute another bad habit when you take away your coping strategy of eating. The goal is to learn how to cope with the emotion using healthy and helpful methods.

One of Larina's favorite rules for handling negative emotions is: *Act in a way opposite to your negative emotion.* When you're depressed, you're tempted to stay in bed all day or eat three plates of lasagna. Do the opposite by getting out and exercising. If you're anxious, you're inclined to avoid the thing that makes you nervous. Do the opposite and confront what you're afraid of; after you've done it several times, you'll gain comfort and confidence. If you're angry, the impulse can be to yell and take it out on someone. Do the opposite by removing yourself from people who could become targets and instead do something nice for someone.

Another useful strategy to make you less likely to succumb to emotional eating is to be sure that you aren't feeling deprived. When people feel deprived of tasty foods, they set themselves up to binge on those foods. When you are overcome by a negative emotion, you're likely to be guided by your feelings and not think rationally, making you more likely to overeat the foods that you crave. Extreme hunger and the feeling that you are deprived make it likely that you'll experience the negative emotion in the first place and that you'll react with emotional eating. Keep yourself nourished to ward off these unruly cravings.

THE BIG EXCUSE

Ready to learn the big excuse that serves to push you down the slippery slope? The major trigger for a backslide is the excuse "I'll eat it *just this time* . . ." Have you ever said this to yourself? Can you see why it can lead to a backslide? Almost any time can be "just this time." This is an excuse that easily snowballs. And once you get into the habit of giving in to excuses, more and more of them creep in.

TIP

Learn to shop smart. Learn to read food labels. Know that foods labeled as "low fat," "low carb," or "dietetic" are frequently mistaken for foods that can be eaten on any diet. It just isn't so. Many foods that are low fat are actually quite high in sugar. Many that are low carb are high in fat and calories. And any food eaten with no regard for portion control is going to make you pack on pounds!

This excuse is often connected to emotional eating. You tell yourself, "I had a really bad day, so I'll have some fettuccine Alfredo *just this time*!" You're enabling your own emotional eating.

The approach that Larina takes to weight loss with her clients is one of moderation, so she typically doesn't recommend that any foods be off limits. As described above, deprivation can lead to overeating, so it is often not a good idea. In the fettuccine Alfredo example, it's not necessarily the food choice (although some foods are obviously healthier than others, so if you choose a highly fattening food like this one, you need to watch the portions very carefully) that's the problem, it's the *reasoning*.

The problem with the "just this time" excuse is that it's an excuse. "Just this time" tends to repeat itself, and before you know it, you're back in an unhealthy eating pattern. Also, according to Larina, the "just this time" excuse tends to put the food in control rather than you in control. It's "that warm chocolate cake is so enticing, I'll just have a piece this time" rather than "I'd love a bit of chocolate so I'll have one bite of my date's dessert." Do you see the difference in who's in control?

If you choose to eat something, take *ownership* for that choice; don't eat in response to your emotions. If, however, you haven't had any chocolate in a while and decide to have a bite of the warm chocolate cake, do it because it will help prevent you from eating a pint of chocolate fudge brownie ice cream later; don't do it because you succumbed to the excuse "just this time." Keep yourself in control. Don't let the food and your excuses gain control.

COOKIE WHIPPED

Victim mentality is a state of mind so easy to fall into when you are caught up in the cycle of weight gain–depression–gain more weight. And complacency is a natural next step. If half the weight-loss battle is in our minds, then shouldn't we just be happy with ourselves, no matter our weight, size, or girth? Maybe that fun-house mirror that puts us in denial when we are at our heaviest—and makes us feel fat even when we have lost weight—is what we should be looking to lose, not the weight!

It's a thought that has recurred for me since I've lost the weight. I've been scrambling to decode whether there is truly a "new" me or whether I'm still the me who always has been. Weight loss causes your mind to churn, and it forces you to reevaluate who you really are, who you were before, and, most important, who you want to be.

People who look at my "before" picture, and then stare at me incredulously, say, "That's not the same person!" And they are right on some level, wrong on other levels. Changes have occurred, no doubt—emotionally, mentally, and physically—but everyone grows and changes. Were the changes because of the weight loss or was the weight loss because of the changes?

The problem is further compounded because frequently others who saw me before didn't really "see" me. Old friends saw a fat, complacently happy housewife who loved to feed and nurture the people around her and who also indulged—OK, *over*indulged—in her own cooking and baking. They didn't know about my problems. I didn't share my feelings. But it's hard to share feelings when you feel victimized, whether your oppressor is a person or an addiction (like food).

People who have never felt victimized—in other words, people with enough self-esteem to be in control of their situations—frequently don't want to hear about it and often can't understand how I got trapped in a situation that I couldn't or refused to control. People tend to shun or further abuse victims. This is why thin people often have a low tolerance for fat people. It is the same with domestic abuse. Even now, after I have conquered my self-esteem problems, I have had people ask me how a smart, savvy, accomplished woman could allow herself to be in an abusive relationship for so long. It's enough to send anyone running to the nearest couch, because the explanation can take a lifetime of self-analysis.

So victims tend *not* to share, not to reach out. They don't want to shoulder more blame; they already have mega-doses of self-blame to deal with. So how do you release your mind from the victim mode?

THE ME LIST

To understand myself better, I made a list. The list reflected not how others saw and see me, but how I saw myself when I was fat and how my *mind* has changed, reflecting the real "new" me:

Old Judy	New Judy	Changes (If Any)
Intelligent	Intelligent	No change
Outspoken	Outspoken	No change
Loving/nurturing	Loving/nurturing	No change
Accomplished	Accomplished	No change
A giver	A giver *and* taker	Change
Weak	Strong and in control	Change

Old Judy	New Judy	Changes (If Any)
Attractive and fat	Attractive, thin, and sexy	Change
Lazy at times	Always in motion	Change
Bleak outlook	The best is yet to come	Change
Dresses frumpy	Dress for success	Change
Abused	No more victim	Huge change
Miserably married	Single	Huge change
Hesitant	Confident	Huge change
Good mother	Better mother	Huge change
Good worker	Excellent worker/supervisor	Huge change

You can make this list at any time during a weight-loss program as a report card on how you are doing. Of course, there will always be room for improvement, but looking back at where you came from and understanding just how far you have come, not just with your weight but also in your life overall, can really keep your mind going in the right direction. It will also give you clarity and enable you to define the benefits of not just the physical aspects of losing weight but the psychological ones as well. Don't rely on smoke and mirrors when you are judging your weight loss. Use concrete tools.

SEVEN

STAYING FIT

Developing Exercise Routines You Can Stick With

WHEN ROSIE GAVE ME THE ONCE-OVER AND IN-formed me that I was an athlete, I was floored. Not only did I never belong to a team in school, but any exercise I ever did as a youth was sporadic and forced. I had no motivation other than the occasional urge to lose a few pounds, and that exercise program would last until the next plate of pasta was winking at me from across the table. The minute I swallowed, I gave up the exercise. I had lapsed into a laconic state, and the very thought of any kind of exercise was sheer torture. To add more "anti-exercise ammunition," an auto accident had put me in traction, with back pain and a slipped disc. I was afraid I would hurt myself more.

ME? AN ATHLETE?

The doctor advised that losing weight would alleviate the pressure on my spine. Yeah—easier said than done! The physical therapists who monitored me suggested that I ease into gentle exercise to strengthen my back. I demurred. Then I began the weight loss. When I hit a plateau, people suggested exercise. That's when I started easing into Pilates. I didn't begin with heavy-duty mat classes. I began one-on-one with a personal trainer, Nancy Adler, who had a neat little Pilates studio with all the equipment—reformer, Cadillac, and barrel—up in her attic. It was costly, but it gave me an entire hour of time—hers and mine—focused on bringing my body into a state of conditioning. It was an investment in my health. When I figured out how much money I had spent on pastries and chocolates over the years, not to mention false starts on various and sundry weight-loss programs, the personal trainer seemed like a good investment.

The other great thing about doing things one-on-one in Nancy's place was that I was sequestered from the intimidating gym scene. I didn't have a bunch of skinny younger girls (or worse, guys) staring at my mounds of flab as they effortlessly jumped around. It was just me and a trusted trainer who was getting to know my body better than I knew it.

If I missed an appointment and didn't give adequate notice, the trainer would charge me anyway. That ensured that I made all my appointments. She was all business, from the moment I walked in until the moment I left. In the beginning, there was very little I could do. My joints were far from limber, my back would spasm, and sometimes during the most gentle exertion, my arrhythmia would kick in and I would have to stop. My trainer knew about all my medical problems, and she knew when not to push me. She took the program at my own pace.

Although my Pilates workouts were plodding along, I was beginning to notice new muscle tone. I was getting stronger, more flexible. I was gradually improving—able to do a little more at each session. I was isolating muscles that I never even knew existed—muscles that had been long buried under piles of fat. The first time Nancy told me to isolate my abdominal muscles, I looked at her weirdly. "There are muscles in there?" I asked her. She laughed. If they were there I sure couldn't feel them, and there was no way I could see them, just rolls and rolls of fat. She explained that they were there, and that if I exercised them, they would help support my back and would likely alleviate the back pain. I began to work on finding the abdominal muscles. It took years, but now I not only feel them, I can see them.

As I continued to lose weight, doing my Pilates religiously once, sometimes twice a week, I began to feel stronger. The pain and cardiac complaints began to abate. There were still some bad days, but most of the time I was able to complete the workout. I also stuck to the weight-loss plan. Then I hit another plateau.

That's when I realized it was time to join a gym. My body was clearly telling me that Pilates wasn't enough. It was time to "shake things up." I joined the local Y and stared at the treadmill in fear. One of the in-house trainers saw me and laughed. When I told her my problems—and that I had never even been on one of these intimidating machines—she guided me to the elliptical machine. "Start with this," she suggested. "It's less rigorous and may be better for your back and knees. You can always move up to the treadmill."

The elliptical became my machine of choice. Once again, I began slowly, twice a week to start, doing a half hour on the elliptical. At first I was short of breath and sweated almost immediately. Slowly my body began getting used to the routine. I extended my workouts to forty minutes and increased the incline and the resistance on the machine. I began to go three times a week, and then four, or sometimes five. Eventually, I found that it took me twenty minutes to break a sweat. I bought wrist weights and scissored my arms in synch with the footwork. I began to switch off from elliptical to treadmill when the exercise became too routine.

There were days when I felt schleppy, ungainly, bloated, or tired; I really didn't want to go to the gym. On those days, I would have to play games with my mind. Sometimes I would take a prayerbook with me on the elliptical and exercise my spiritual being along with my physical one. Other days I would pretend to be a secret agent in training. I would work up a creative scenario in which the world was depending on me to defend my country. The treadmill would become a battlefield filled with land mines that I had to navigate to free my platoon. The imaginative games made the workout fun and I would throw myself into them as if human life depended on me. At least one did—my own!

It was physics 101: a body in motion yearned to stay in motion.

The more I exercised, the better I felt. Not just because my clothes were fitting better and I was getting compliments, but because when I neglected to exercise, I really felt the difference. My moods would change. I would feel more stressed. Emotionally I was becoming "addicted" to the good feeling I got after a workout. I can't live without that good feeling for any length of time now. I can't imagine how I lived without it beforehand.

The trainers in the gym watched in amazement as I got thinner. My gym clothes went from big T-shirts to baggy T-shirts to sleek spandex that showed off my newfound curves. I added belly-dancing classes, jujitsu, and, recently, kickboxing. I suddenly realized that I'm no longer intimidated by a gym full of toned and fit men and women.

And, here's the thing: While I can always find someone

in the kickboxing class who is more toned, more fit, has better endurance, is younger (or older and spunkier!) than me, it doesn't matter. Some have thin ropey muscles, others are heavy; some are waiflike and delicate, others are a combination of muscle and fat. I look and I learn. But I'm no longer intimidated. Because getting fit is not a race or competition; rather, it is about health and fun and making the most of every minute of my workout. And walking away feeling great, physically and emotionally.

And guess what? I *am* an athlete!

WHY YOU *NEED* TO EXERCISE

Since you've successfully lost weight, it's likely that you are familiar with a lifestyle that incorporates exercise. While this physical activity was beneficial in helping you lose the weight, it wasn't enough. Typically, exercise plus nutritional changes produce weight loss. Exercise serves as a great adjunct to your dietary changes. Research by the National Institutes of Health and the National Heart, Lung and Blood Institute indicates that diet or diet plus exercise generally produces greater weight loss than exercise by itself.

Most of us who have lost weight and managed to keep it off have learned to love exercise—or at least love the results it brings. How important is exercise *now* that the weight is gone?

Very important. The most important role of exercise is not in the weight-loss phase but in the maintenance of weight loss. Research shows that those who stick to an exercise regimen are most likely to stay in The Thin Club. Regular exercise is a good predictor of keeping weight off.

The National Weight Control Registry tracked people who successfully maintained their weight loss over 5.5

years. They found that only 9 percent reported maintaining their weight *without* regular physical activity. This means that 91 percent of those who were able to keep their weight off engaged in regular activity, typically a combination of lifestyle and programmed exercise. Likewise, results of a three-year study of men showed that those who exercised showed better long-term weight loss compared with those who only dieted. That shouldn't come as a surprise, but get this: If exercise was added during the follow-up period, weight was either lost or maintained, but diet alone resulted in steady weight gain. So *only* changing your eating habits after you have lost weight can lead to weight regain.

TIP

Breathe! Seems like a given, but when you're keyed up and anxious, you tend to hold your breath. Letting it out while you're exercising will circulate the oxygen and give you more energy and stamina during a workout. It is a great way to keep yourself going when you feel like you just can't do one more leg lift!

Larina believes that exercise is so vitally important because of its mental, not physical, benefit. There are obviously tons of physical benefits, but the most important mental benefit is that exercise keeps your mind toned. When you work out, you are reminding yourself that health and fitness are strong values that you are choosing to live by. Because exercise is immediately rewarding, owing to the feel-good hormones that are stimulated, you receive a reward for doing something good for yourself. According to bariatric expert Dr. J. Shah, during or after exercise our bodies secrete good hormones (such as growth hormone, estrogen, progesterone, testosterone, insulin, endorphins, thyroid, and insulin) as well as glucagons. These all have beneficial effects on the body's metabolism. Additionally, the hormone level of cortisol goes down, which benefits the body for weight loss. Thus, exercise keeps you in the mindset of health. This mindset can guarantee you lifetime membership in The Thin Club.

TIP

After you exercise, draw extra attention to the positive mental benefits of the exercise by writing them down. For example, you may say, "I am practicing what I preach about the importance of health and fitness." Or, "My mind is clear and sharp whenever I leave a great spinning class," or "I am committed to staying in shape and it feels great to exercise."

Exercise is also helpful in keeping calories in perspective. Let's say that you've just completed an intense cardiovascular workout: 45 minutes on the treadmill. Upon completion of your workout, the treadmill screen says that you've burned 300 calories. You feel great! As you're pulling out of the parking lot, out of the corner of your eye you see a sign for your favorite bagel bakery. You aren't really hungry, but the idea of a big, doughy Cheddar-scallion bagel with cream cheese is very tempting. But, wait, you think—how many calories are in that big bagel and topping? Around 400! If you ate it, you would pull out of that parking lot with a net *gain* of 100 calories after your intense workout! Is it worth it? No, you decide, it's definitely not. You decide to wait for your healthy dinner later in the evening.

TIP

Without becoming obsessive, pay attention to the calories in food and how much exercise it takes to burn them off. If three bites of rich ice cream can cost you 100 calories, ask yourself whether you have the time or desire to burn an extra 100 calories in the gym today. You may decide that those bites of ice cream just aren't worth it.

WHAT KIND OF EXERCISE TO DO

OK, now that you are convinced to keep up with your exercise program, you're probably wondering what type of exercise is the best to do and how much. According to research and the experts, strength training seems to be an important component in the exercise programs of those who keep weight off.

Rob Zschau, a personal trainer and corporate/personal wellness consultant in the St. Louis area, with fifteen years of experience in the fitness and wellness industry, says that an effective exercise schedule should include cardiovascular exercise, resistance training, and muscle building. Cardiovascular exercise, he adds, is the only way to burn fat in the largest amounts and safest manner possible. Used in conjunction with proper eating, he says, it is the most efficient way to get rid of saddlebags and other fat deposits on the body. Resistance training, he stresses, gives the underlying muscle and fat shape so that what is left after you lose the weight is (we hope) nice to look at.

Muscle building also plays a role in how much fat your body burns when you are doing cardio. The more muscle you have, the more fat you burn doing cardio and throughout the entire day. Basic maintenance after a successful weight loss should include at least three days a week of cardio exercise (walking, bike, elliptical) for thirty minutes (but a maximum of one hour) inside your target heart rate, which will be between 55 percent and 85 percent of your estimated maximum heart rate. If you're not sure how to figure it out, ask a qualified personal trainer to help you.

A much higher proportion of registered subjects in the National Weight Control Registry reported performing regular resistance training compared with the general population. Research shows that resistance exercise may prevent weight gain or regain. This is because resistance exercise keeps your resting metabolic rate and lean body mass elevated. This means less fat and more calorie burning even when you're just sitting around. But you don't need to spend hours each day exercising. Fortunately, frequent activity at a moderately intense level can be as effective as longer exercise sessions less often.

HOW MUCH EXERCISE TO DO

The next obvious question is "How much physical activity is needed to minimize weight regain in previously overweight individuals?" The answer may surprise you. It's actually necessary to be active at a moderate to high level of intensity almost every day. You may not like this, but as you know, there is no quick and easy fix or substitute for a healthy lifestyle that leads to weight loss or keeping weight off. For those of you thinking of your busy schedules and wondering how you're going to fit in exercise every day, rest assured that you will not need to do hours each day.

One research team found that formerly obese women who were successful at maintaining their weight loss for one year participated in approximately 80 minutes a day of moderate-intensity activity or 35 minutes a day of vigorous activity. You must expend around 2,500 calories per week to maintain weight loss.

TIP

Save yourself some time by turning your exercise intensity up a notch. Many exercise machines will tell you whether you are in the optimal intensity zone for fat burning. If you do your cardiovascular exercise outdoors (which is great since it can provide beautiful, motivating scenery), first spend some time practicing with exercise equipment to get a sense of the right level of intensity. Then mimic it with your outdoors activities.

So, what does this mean? It means that if you are serious about maintaining your Thin Club membership, you need to get moving, nearly every day! This includes formal and informal exercise, so going up and down the stairs at work and walking your dog does count! Of course, if you are careful about regulating your eating, you can get away without exercising every day, but exercise is a major player in keeping your new, post-weight-loss body.

MOTION MOTIVATION

TIP

Mentally motivate yourself by focusing on all the wonderful things that have resulted from your commitment to exercise. Remind yourself that you'll have to keep up with the exercise routine to reap the physical and emotional benefits of becoming fit. Think of the exercise as having helped you reach your goal and be thankful for it—it is a great ally to you. Now that you've met your goal, don't forget the things that helped you get there!

Getting out the door on kickboxing nights (or mornings) isn't always easy, even though I *know* I have to and I know how great I'll feel afterward. For me, it is the "before" that I find most challenging. Once I've taken the plunge—made the effort to get to the gym, track, or on the balance ball—I can usually convince myself to make the most of my workout. And halfway through I may even resist looking at the clock. But getting there is half the battle. It's sometimes too cold, too hot, I have aches, I'm too tired. But I have found that what I learned in high school physics was true: A body in motion *does* tend to stay in motion. Getting started is the key.

When you were losing weight, you were probably very motivated by your goal and loved watching the pounds come off. Now that you're living in a thinner body, you need to look to some other things to keep you motivated. If you're loving life in the thinner body, that in itself can motivate you. Keep yourself keenly aware of all the enjoyable aspects of life as a fit person. When you go up a couple flights of stairs without becoming winded, bask in the feeling of accomplishment. When you notice your toned muscles after a great session of resistance training, remember that feeling to help you get back to the gym the next time.

One life coach and personal fitness trainer, also a bodybuilder (a former Mr. San Diego), shared that he motivates himself by always putting himself first. "I may seem selfish," he explains, "but if I take care of my own needs, I know that I can be there for anybody. I'll be a better son, a better boyfriend, I'll be better with my clients and better overall. So I selfishly push myself to work out." And that propels him to the gym every day, whether he is tired, achy, or just plain not in the mood. Nothing disrupts his routine.

Staying motivated to exercise is a constant challenge, especially to keep up with the intensity and frequency that we are recommending. What are some of the things Thin Club members do to keep themselves in motion?

TIP

Losing motivation during an exercise class? Give yourself an internal challenge! Instead of giving up and flopping on the floor like everyone else during the final eight push-ups, give that last set the very best effort you can, remembering that you won't be doing this for a while. Each additional push-up is one more bite of something you ate yesterday, sweating out of your pores! So while you're on the floor, make that last count "count"!

TELL A FRIEND!

You've probably heard about how helpful it is to have a workout buddy. This is because you can help motivate each other to stick to your plans. If one of you is low on energy and ready to bail out of the Rollerblading session you'd planned, the other can help motivate to do it anyway.

Stephanie Rhodes was a diet-book groupie for most of her life. She owns dozens of diet books and has tried every diet, but she has gained the weight back each time. She has started exercise programs only to find herself loathing the thought of working out. It wasn't until she played a game that her daughter Vicki invented that she found the motivation to exercise on a regular basis and keep her weight off.

The idea of the game was to create a friendly eight-week exercise competition with two people (she invented it to get her and her fiancé in shape for their wedding). The only way to win the game was to exercise at least three times a week for the entire eight weeks. When she first played it, she found that having a partner holding her accountable, as well as the competitive aspect of the game, really gave her the much-needed motivation to stay with the program. Both she and Vicki lost weight and kept it off.

Three years later, Stephanie has adopted exercise as part of her daily life, walking four miles every morning. It has led her to better eating habits and an overall healthy lifestyle, leading her to keep weight off. As a believer in her daughter's creation, Stephanie became a business partner with Vicki and together they brought the idea to market. Naming the game The Fitness Challenge, they have heard from hundreds of people who have played it, helping them to incorporate exercise into their overall weight-loss program. Visit her website www.fitnesschallenge.com

if you would like to take advantage of Stephanie's tips and join the challenge!

TIP

Use games to make it fun. While you do your dips and chin-ups on the Gravitron or run on the treadmill, picture yourself in your post-workout shape—but take it a step further. Imagine your buff self running up a mountain, perhaps doing something extraordinary to save the world, your family, or your neighborhood from the evil empire. You are the hero who tackles Osama bin Laden, the quarterback with just the right form to make the winning throw, whatever. . . . Use your imagination to workout harder, even if you're doing it by yourself! Or, steal a look at the guy or gal next to you. Challenge yourself to be better, stronger, stay on longer than that person! Now, the workout gets interesting!

Do not wait to be motivated to exercise. Think about it. If you are exhausted after a long day of work, enjoying a great movie or TV program, trying to catch up on all your errands, or relaxing with a good book, of course you won't be motivated to exercise. There will almost always be something else to do.

TIP

Act first, motivate second. Remember that once you start exercising, you will likely become more motivated. It's always the beginning that's the hardest, so the key is to get yourself in motion even without motivation. The

motivation will come, especially if you picked an enjoyable exercise routine.

One of the most important parts of having an exercise
buddy is holding one another accountable. If your friend is
planning to pick you up at 7 P.M. to head off to the gym together, you'll get yourself ready so you don't disappoint or
inconvenience her. It's much easier to cancel plans with
yourself than with someone else.

If you don't have a workout partner, you have a couple
of choices: You can get one, or you can work on a system
to hold yourself accountable. To get a partner, ask friends
and friends of friends, family members, and anyone else
you can think of. You can also begin your exercise activities solo and meet people. For example, one of Larina's
clients became a regular in a Pilates class and also in a
cardio-kickboxing class. She decided to enjoy the social aspect of the classes along with the great exercise, so she introduced herself and chatted with different people who
regularly attended the class. She met a woman who lived a
couple of blocks from her and they decided to carpool to
the gym three times a week and share babysitting. They
were able to hire one babysitter for both sets of kids, so
they saved money on babysitting and gas and were able to
ensure regular workouts.

TIP

*If it's hard to motivate yourself, work on motivating your
workout friend.* Give each other compliments and support. Come up with a workout routine that works for
both of you. Anticipate all the things that could get in

the way of sticking to the routine and problem-solve together.

TRICK YOURSELF

To motivate yourself, come up with a way to hold yourself accountable. You can write your exercise schedule on a calendar on your refrigerator and cross off each activity that you attend and circle everything that you don't attend with a big red marker. You'll be motivated to keep those red circles off your calendar.

You can also try tricks, such as going right from work to the gym before any excuses can get in the way; you have to visit the gym, like putting something that you'll need in your locker. You may have found some good tricks that worked for you while you were losing weight; don't forget about them now that you've lost the weight—they may help you stay motivated now.

TIP

Make an emergency motivation-music mix. There are some songs that always pump us up. These are the songs that you cannot help but to smile when you hear them. They bring up your energy level and mood. When you need an instant energy and inspiration fix to get going, play these tunes and get moving!

So don't wait to get motivated or inspired. You could be waiting for a long time—so long that your Thin Club membership could expire.

TIP

Buy exercise clothes that flatter! OK, so no one looks really glam in workout clothes—at least not in the kind of heavy-duty workout clothes that are likely to stay on during an intense and sweaty workout. Still, buy the best-fitting, nicest style of workout clothes you can—oversized T-shirts and baggy sweats just won't cut it! And watch yourself in the mirror as you flex those newly formed muscles. Take pride in what you have become and are becoming. At the gym, enjoy being a work-in-progress!

CAN WE REALLY CHANGE OUR SHAPE?

All of us are born with a certain number of fat cells, and when we are very young, these cells divide and multiply. At some point (doctors can't agree on exactly when and how it is determined), the cells stop dividing and we are left with the number of fat cells we will carry around forever—and they deposit themselves wherever they may cluster. There are two primary fat-distribution patterns: the android "apple" shape, with more upper-body fat, more commonly found in men, and the gynoid "pear" shape, commonly found in women. The distribution pattern is largely dependent on genetics, but there are some environmental factors. If we yo-yo diet, we tend to accumulate more upper-body fat. And as we age, the distribution pattern can change. Some fat cells surround and coat our internal organs as "cushioning." Other fat cells are closer to the surface of our skin. And all of our fat cells have the capacity to inflate with lipids when we feed them and deflate when we diet and exercise.

THE BODY MASS INDEX

You may notice after a rigorous workout that you actually look slimmer. Is this an optical illusion or reality? Fat cells will shrink when you diet and exercise, but they will never go away naturally. Surgical procedures like liposuction can remove external layers of fat, but fat cells around your organs—the ones that really threaten your health—can never be removed. The only way to control them is through diet.

Is there an objective way to know if you are "still fat" after all that diet and exercise? The answer is yes. While you may find yourself still quite subjectively fat when you look in a mirror, hop on a scale, or compare your muscles, bones, and waist measurement to impossibly thin actresses on the cover of *People* magazine, or you lust endlessly after a smaller size dress, Body Mass Index (BMI) is the definitive test. For the mathematicians among us, BMI equals your weight in pounds/height in inches^2 x 703. That means a person who weighs 220 pounds and is 6 foot 3 inches tall has a BMI of 27.5. A person who weighs 134 pounds and is 5 foot 7 inches tall has a BMI of 21. So, to figure out if you are technically fat or technically thin, just do the math and see where you fall into the table below:

BMI	WEIGHT STATUS
Below 18.5	Underweight
18.5–24.9	Normal
25.0–29.9	Overweight
30.0 and Above	Obese

That said, BMI is not the sole indicator of health and wellness, and while it is a good indicator, it doesn't measure body fat. A bodybuilder with major muscle mass could theoretically have the same BMI as a person who doesn't work out and has a higher ratio of fat to muscle. To determine the percentage of fat, you need calipers or a special electronic scale. The calipers pinch the skin of the triceps, biceps, subscapula (fold just below the shoulder blade), or suprailiac (just above the hip bone); based on how many millimeters are pinched, there are tables to determine fat-to-muscle ratio. Most gyms and weight-loss centers can help you do this.

When you begin or increase your level of exercise and resistance training, you may be frustrated that pounds on the scale do not budge. This is because you are changing your body composition. As you lose fat, you build muscle. Because of this, most health and fitness researchers say that body composition (percentage of fat and muscle) is a much more important indicator of health than weight.

While a pound of muscle does not weigh more than a pound of fat (both weigh a pound, right?), muscle is more dense than fat and fat takes up more room. When you begin losing fat and replacing it with muscle, you'll lose size and take up less space, but you may not lose weight. Fat cells are less dense than muscle cells because fat cells contain mostly oils while muscle cells contain mostly proteins and water. Oils are less dense than water (think about what happens when you mix water and oil—the oil goes up to the top). The lowered density of fatty tissue makes it less heavy than muscle.

CAN I REALLY LOSE MY BELLY, LOVE HANDLES, ARM FLAB, ETC.?

There is no way for anyone to know what areas of the body are going to spring back or not after a massive weight loss (or even a slight one). The factors that lead up to how the body will react to weight loss include many things, such as how much weight is lost, how fast it is lost, where most of the fat accumulated on the body, whether male or female, age, genes, and skin tightness, just to name a few. All of these factors and more make it impossible to know just how the body will do after weight loss. However, the average person should see good toning and an overall positive body look after losing weight and beginning exercise.

WHEN TO WORK OUT/HOW TO FUEL

Time is on your side, no matter what time of day you decide to work out. It is more important that you show up and do it than to worry about when the best time of day is to work out. Work out at whatever time of day is best for you. And it's important to fuel up before *and* after a workout. "Eating a little food about an hour before will give you the energy you need to sustain your body through a workout," explains trainer Rob Zschau. "It also helps prevent bad things from happening, like low blood sugar. When you are finished with your workout you need to take in some more food—not necessarily a whole meal, although that would be all right."

Cynthia Sass, a dietitian and the coauthor of *Your Diet Is Driving Me Crazy: When Food Conflicts Get in the Way of Your Love Life,* and an expert on nutrition and sports, explains that while the body will burn body fat during a workout, it will also burn glycogen reserves that are stored in the muscles. If you run out of glycogen you will eat away at the protein part of the muscle; therefore, eating adequately and eating enough healthy carbs provide adequate glycogen levels, which are used as fuel during exercise.

"Foods that are difficult to digest—high protein, high-fiber, and fatty foods—delay the emptying of the stomach. These should be avoided two hours before exercising so that you can maximize the energy and be comfortable during your workout. Optimal pre-workout foods include low-fiber, complex carbohydrate foods like yogurt, half an English muffin with a no-sugar-added fruit spread, or a small baggie of Kix or Cheerios." She recommends the following basic diets for the following workouts:

- **Heavy-Strength Training** To build muscle mass, you require a slightly higher protein intake. One gram of protein per pound of body weight is slightly over what a strength-training athlete needs, but it should promote muscle building.
- **Endurance** Running, aerobic exercise, or my favorite, kickboxing, require that at least 50 percent of calories come from low-glycemic carbohydrates. High-fiber fruits are OK because of their essential nutrients.
- **Flexibility** To promote joint health and discourage inflammation, eat plant-based oils, olive oil, and vegetable oil, as well as flaxseed, nuts, and fatty fish.

FIND THE RIGHT GYM

Gyms can be intimidating, especially if you've been out of the scene for a while. Before joining a facility, map out the gyms closest to you and find out which are affordable. The closer the gym, the fewer excuses you will have for missing a day.

Visit the facility at the time of day you are most likely to exercise and take in the ambience. Is the facility appealing? Does it appear to be clean? Is it a place that you could see yourself spending time? Is the décor soothing, energizing, challenging—and how does it make you feel? Do the gym members appear to interact or do you get a serious "leave me alone" attitude from them? Is there an uncomfortable competitive feeling in the room? Are the other members close to your own age? These are all factors that could make or break your gym experience (and cause you to fall off the wagon if they aren't right from the get-go).

Does the gym offer a wide variety of classes for every level of fitness? While you may be starting out on one level, half a year later you may be several levels ahead. Will the facility accommodate the "new you"? Note whether all the machines are in use. If some are not, check to see if they are operational. Also, watch the trainers who supervise the exercise room. Are they interacting with the gym members, helping them with the machines? Do they seem to pay attention to some while ignoring others? Do they seem preoccupied with phone calls, gossiping with other staff members, or reading magazines? Ask your tour guide whether the trainers are paid to help out customers who need to learn the equipment or are there simply for one-on-one (paid) sessions.

Audit an exercise class. How crowded is the room? Do you have enough room to really spread out, or is someone invading your personal space? Are there enough exercise accessories for everyone in the class? Does anyone seem left out when the instructor goes around to check on the students' "form" during the class?

Are small children allowed in the room during exercise classes? Common sense dictates that children should be cared for in a separate room while the parents are exercising. There is nothing more disconcerting than having a small child running behind you as you are kicking, punching, dancing, or otherwise focused on an active workout. If you want to make exercise a family event, find programs specifically geared to the whole family. It's a great way to make your family fit and trim along with you. Many Y's have family swims, hiking and biking events, even adventure trips that families can enjoy together.

Some gyms are "male dominated," and if you are female, this can lead to inequity and even sexual harassment. If you suspect the gym might be male oriented, but you are interested in that particular type of exercise, check the cancellation policy before you sign up and try a short-term contract before committing to more long-term membership, regardless of cost savings. This trial membership can save you an unpleasant experience and potential loss of money down the line.

TIP

Get seven to eight hours of sleep each night. Sleep deprivation makes you more susceptible to stress and negative emotions, which lead to emotional eating. We're also less likely to pay attention to what we eat when we're exhausted, and we end up overeating. And if that's not enough to convince you, there's now evidence that people who are sleep deprived have reduced levels of the hormone leptin. Low levels of leptin increase feelings of hunger and overeating. Instead of falling prey to sleep-related problems, prioritize your sleep to help you keep your Thin Club membership!

PART TWO

WHO
AM
I?

Living Life

as

"The New You"

EIGHT

FRIENDS AND FOES

Developing a Positive
Support Network

IT WASN'T SO LONG AGO WHEN I WAS THE ONE being sniped at for taking up one and a half seats in a commuter train. So why do I sometimes find myself watching a heavy person and feeling not empathy but disgust? Someone confronted me in a dating site chat room: "Judy, you've shared your weight-loss story with us, so why do you refuse to date anyone who is overweight?" He is right. My profile read: "Looking for someone who takes pride in his appearance—that means choosing Green Tea over Dunkin' Donuts!" And I meant every word of it. I've become a bit of a weight-loss crusader. Does that make me a bitch? Some might say yes.

AM I A BITCH?

Can a fat person really be friends with someone thin? Can a thin person look at a fat person without judging, blaming, pitying the person's lack of self-control? The fat issue is so much bigger than food choices and activity levels. When we choose to be thin, we are choosing more than the right foods. We are choosing long-term health over ephemeral flavor. We are choosing willpower and self-control over helplessness and structure over impulse.

Hollywood and Broadway embrace the fat-thin friendship ideal. Laurel and Hardy, Abbott and Costello, The Odd Couple, Lucy and Ethel, Lorelai Gilmore and Sookie, Raven and Chelsea—you get the picture. Frequently the fat characters exemplify helpless, unstructured foodaholics while the thin ones are control freaks. But when we get beyond the stereotypes, are there inherent relationship challenges to a fat-thin friendship?

I made friends with Cindy long before I lost all the weight and years before my divorce. She became a food buddy. We would spend long, lazy afternoons munching on home-baked goodies, watching videos, and creating recipes that were anything but healthy. Equal opportunity foodies, we enjoyed the gamut of gourmet, homestyle, and comfort cuisine. We talked about everything—our imperfect marriages, our angst over our kids, our disgust with our burgeoning bodies, our aches and pains. We would go out to bars and share an occasional "girl's night out" beer, sometimes with other friends who were, like myself, on the cusp of or sometimes over the edge of morbidly obese.

We had plenty to say about those size 4 neighborhood cuties who ate a rice cake as a meal and exercised as if their lives depended on it. They never had to worry about their weight. Of course, they were naturally slender. We rolled our eyes and scoffed at their perfect bodies and their presumably perfect lives. These women were a different breed from "real women" like us. They had everything a woman could want: great husbands and lots of money that they didn't have to earn themselves, and they didn't look their age. And even if they did, they could fix that with a quick operation. They had plenty of time to care for themselves, not like us.

And then I got thin. Of course, it was gradual, and we all started out dieting together. Cindy and I stuck to it the longest, while our other friends dropped out early in the game. Then she had an upset in her life, and one day I came into her kitchen to pick her up for our thrice-weekly power walk and found her picking apart a loaf of crusty semolina bread as she drained a bottle of pinot noir. It was carb comfort at its best.

"Do you really want to wreck it all?" I asked her gently. "You were doing so well."

"Don't *ever* tell me what to do, Ms. Perfect Know-it-all," she snapped at me. "I hate when people tell me what to eat. My mother used to do that all the time, and it drove me nuts. I'll get back to the diet when I'm ready."

I backed out of the kitchen, far away from the bread knife that was still slicing through the loaf of bread as Cindy stuffed her face with gobs of gluten in her two-fisted effort to regain every pound she had worked so hard to lose. Our power walks soon stalled and I joined a gym to maintain my cardio workout. Cindy and I stopped seeing each other as often as we had. The next time I saw her she had put on about fifty pounds. I had lost another ten. She was going through a bag of Oreos along with our old gang of food girls. Cindy didn't seem thrilled to see me, and she put the cookies down as I walked in.

"Don't you look great," she said in a forced tone. "You're so skinny. Isn't she skinny, girls?" There were nods of agreement.

"You're really keeping it off! But isn't that neckline kind of low, don't you think? Is it really appropriate for someone our age to walk around looking . . . well . . ."

"Sexy?" I finished her sentence.

"It's just that we are women of a certain age," she said defensively. The other women in the room smirked in agreement. Ouch!

"Can I get you anything? Tea? I'd offer you cookies," she pointed at the half-empty Oreo package, "but I already know the answer to that one. . . ."

And then I realized. I had inadvertently switched sides. I had become the enemy—one of the slender Thin Club members who ate a rice cake for lunch. The ones I used to scoff at with my former posse. I was no longer Cindy's munchy, crunchy food friend. I was in the middle of my divorce, and if ever I needed my girlfriends to download to, it was then. But I knew there was no sympathy in that house. Quite the contrary, the room would be buzzing when I left, with them probably bashing me because of my impending divorce and because I was dressing sexier. My life was changing, and while I did not miss our apoplectic food-fests, I missed the Cindy I used to talk to about everything. Now, more than ever, I needed someone to walk and talk with me. What had happened?

In some of my old circles, I had been the subject of rumors from the day I started looking and dressing better. The day I announced I was leaving my husband, the neighborhood was in an uproar.

"I knew it." Husbands were nudging their wives, some obviously scared. "She got thin and sexy and she left him!" All true. I did. And to some, I became public enemy number one. If it could happen to me, it could happen to them. Some neighbors actually walked by me, noses in the air, refusing to say hello. Divorce frequently breaks up friendships, but divorce after someone has gotten thin and changed appearance causes endless speculation and some biting, nasty attitudes.

Little by little, I began to make new friends—not always thin, but frequently more body conscious, athletic, and with more self-pride than the friends I used to have. The women I befriended post-weight-loss didn't feel out of control, overwhelmed or controlled by food, or have the need to disdain other women who took time for themselves or to care for their bodies. It seemed like people were falling into two categories: those who had self-image problems and those with positive self-images. It was those in The Fat Club and those in The Thin Club—and it wasn't size that made the difference. It was their attitude. These days, I choose The Thin Club.

SEPARATING FRIEND-IN-NEED FROM FOE INDEED

Once you are part of The Thin Club, will all your friendships survive? If you are already in The Thin Club, how are people helping or sabotaging your membership? Support for your weight-loss efforts is monumentally important. In Larina's model of weight loss, called STRENGTH Weight Loss & Wellness, one of the eight components of losing weight and keeping it off is Support (the *S* in the word *strength;* see www.StrengthWeightLoss.com for a free e-course that mentions the others). You can lose weight without support, but it is hard. You can keep it off without support, but that is even harder.

You may try to be strong and think you don't need the support of others. But don't fool yourself. And don't make your weight loss harder than it needs to be. Plus, when you have a great support system, the whole process becomes more fun and you feel good that you are able to help others as well.

To get support that will truly help you, you need to

surround yourself with the right types of people. As you go through the process of losing weight and maintaining your goal weight, you need to ask yourself the important and difficult question: Who's a friend and who's a foe? To answer this question, you take an honest look at your relationships and decide who's supporting you and who's sabotaging you.

Are there ways to preserve the friendships in spite of potential jealousy on their part, attitude changes you've made, and changes in the equilibrium of your friendship? Yes. But you'll have to think carefully about how to do this and what you want.

OLD FRIENDS, NEW PERSPECTIVES

Here's a multiple-choice quiz to help you.

1. Most of my friendships have been:
   a. Based around eating.
   b. Generally supportive with some mild jealousy and competitiveness.
   c. Very supportive of me regardless of my situation.

2. If I'm feeling down and I go to a friend's house, she is most likely to say:
   a. "Let's drown it in hot fudge!"
   b. "But you have so much going for you—you're thin now!'
   c. "Let's talk about it over a brisk hike."

3. Regarding my new look, I believe my friends:
   a. Are mostly envious and they assume I've changed inside as well.
   b. Slightly jealous, but very proud and supportive.

    c. Very proud, supportive, encouraging, and
       helpful.

4. If I go out to eat with my friends now that I am
   thinner, I feel:
    a. Uncomfortable, scrutinized and judged.
    b. A little uncomfortable when the food comes if
       I'm the only one eating something healthy.
    c. Very confident and comfortable—we're focused
       on each other, not on the food.

5. If I wanted to talk with friends about the challenges
   I'm going through as I lose weight and try to keep it
   off, I'd feel:
    a. That they wouldn't understand because they'd
       be consumed with thinking of themselves.
    b. That they would listen and try to be helpful
       even though they don't understand and may feel
       envious.
    c. That they would listen and provide continuous
       support and encouragement in a nonjudgmental
       and helpful manner.

FORMER FOOD BUDDIES

If you answered with mostly *A*s, your friends are likely to be former food buddies. These are fair-weather friends who stick around when donuts and pizza are in the forecast. They are likely to be overweight or have low self-esteem themselves and to project their difficulties onto you. They feel threatened by your new appearance, your success, energy, and vitality. If you are sure that *you* have not changed your behavior in a negative way, then you can be sure that these friends are more like foes.

The problem with these friendships is that they were

based on one aspect of your existence (eating), rather than on you as a whole person. If a friend or spouse is only able to support you if there are double fudge brownies involved, the person is *not supportive*. One of the most important aspects of a friendship is the ability to listen empathically with positive regard for the friend. If a friend becomes judgmental, consumed with his or her jealousy and concerns about his or her own appearance, or sets up an us (fat) versus them (thin) situation to ostracize you, then it may be time to lose 190 more pounds (your friend!).

Another difficulty with spending time with former food buddies is that you are going to be more likely to put yourself in situations that lead to unhealthy eating. If eating junk food was a major basis of your friendship, unhealthy situations are likely to present themselves again. This is not to say that you must cut ties with all heavy people! If, however, all of the activities these former food buddies want to do center on going to all-you-can-eat buffets, you'll need to proceed with caution. Plus, if these friends are making comments that put you on the defensive and create discomfort and stress, you will be more likely to slip into emotional eating and make unhealthy choices.

First, try to be highly assertive with these friends to see if they are capable of meeting your needs. When your friend Sam suggests drowning your sorrows in hot fudge, you can say, "Sam, you know how hard I've worked on changing my emotional eating patterns. I'd love to have your support if we can do it without food."

Next, state what you need from your friend. Give it several tries and use the broken-record technique by saying the same response each time your friend is unhelpful. If the friend isn't getting it and appears to be insensitive or, worse, sabotaging your efforts, then it's time to break the friendship. If it's a friendship that you valued and hope will resume someday, then you may want to be honest with your friend about why you need time apart.

UNSURE FRIENDS

If you answered mostly *Bs*, then you have friends who want to be supportive but are unsure how to be. They may have their own insecurities about their weight. They might feel uncomfortable around you because it makes them feel inadequate that they haven't lost the weight. This is not your fault. While your friends may be struggling with their own issues, they are likely to be ones who do care about you and want to support you.

You may need to educate these friends about how to be around you. They may feel like they are making a mistake by suggesting that you meet for lunch. Or they may worry that you want to surround yourself with others in The Thin Club and that they will lose you as a friend. The best way to handle this situation is to be upfront and open with your friends.

Sometimes people do not support others simply because they don't know how to. This comes up in all sorts of ways. For example, often women feel unsupported by their husbands because their husbands try to solve the problem without listening to the situation. When a wife tells her husband that she is best supported by empathic listening rather than problem solving, he can keep that in mind to best offer support. So, begin by telling your friend what you'd like now that you are working toward an important goal of weight loss or maintenance.

You can also look for ways to support your friends as they grapple with their own problems that were brought up by your weight loss. If you want support, the best thing you can do is give support. Your friends may feel sad and like failures because you were able to lose weight and they haven't. This idea can hold true for thin friends as well. Your thin friends may be trying to achieve an important undertaking and feel plagued by the thought "Sally could lose ninety pounds and I can't even do this one small thing!"

Remember that some jealousy is normal and expected. The envy itself is not so much a problem as is the way in which your friends express it or make you feel guilty. We're all a bit envious of different aspects of different people's lives. The best ways to help yourself end making assumptions is to suspend your own judgment and check things out with your friends before you create fables in your mind.

It's also important not to assume. You may feel pressured to order dessert, assuming that your friend will conclude that you're a thin snob if you don't, whereas in reality your friend could care less if you order dessert.

But what about when people are critical of you? Or when even you are critical about yourself because of how you lost the weight? This sounds bizarre but it happens! One of Larina's clients, Sara, was moving her way down the scale when she became frustrated by how people responded to her main method of weight loss: her eating. People were critical and skeptical about the 180-degree turnaround Sara had done with her eating. Once addicted to chips, fast food, and chocolate shakes, Sara developed a healthy obsession with organic, natural foods. She truly enjoyed her newfound commitment to healthy eating and having a well-balanced diet. She took vitamin supplements, avoided gluten and white sugar, and ate tons of organic fruits and veggies. "You're obsessed!" people told her, "You need to lighten up!"

Well, lightening up (her weight) was just Sara's intent.

But she felt scrutinized and criticized as she became committed to her new way of eating, and felt like people thought she could do nothing right. Interestingly, people used to give her disgusted looks when she'd eat huge amounts of greasy food, but no one said anything. Now, people seemed to feel justified to say, "Stop reading the food labels all the time—you're skinny now."

People often have a hard time adjusting to change. Whether it is change in themselves or in someone else, change is often stressful. They were used to you as the fast-food, french-fry girl who ate spontaneously anything in front of her. They aren't used to you now that you're a thoughtful eater who takes time to read labels and ask questions about what to order at a restaurant. These are changes that others must adjust to. Help them to do so. But if they can't, you may have to consider spending less time with people who are critical in an unsupportive way.

TIP

Educate others about your new habits. People are often critical about that which they don't understand. Let them know about your goals, habits, and new behaviors and request their support.

SUPPORTIVE FRIENDS

If you answered mostly *C*s, you're lucky! You have some highly supportive friends. These are deep friendships that transcend the number of pounds you carry around. These are the friends who will love you if you're fat or thin, young or old, happy or sad. Realize that these are ideal friendships, but most friendships in reality are not ideal.

Many of your friendships will contain a mix of supportiveness and uncertainty.

The support of these friends is going to help you remain in The Thin Club. It's up to you to use the support they're offering you. Of course, there's a fine line between requesting too little support and too much. You don't want to underutilize your friends because then you will miss the benefits of having friends to do enjoyable activities with, keep you motivated to make healthy eating and exercise decisions, and help you stay on track. On the other hand, you don't want to overtap these friends, leaving them feeling burned out. Be sure that you are supporting them as much as they are supporting you.

TIP

What kinds of friends do you have? Take a close look at who falls into which of the categories listed above. If the biggest part of your friendship equates to a deep-dish pizza with some of your friends, you may need to separate yourself to ensure your membership in The Thin Club.

NEW YOU, NEW FRIENDS

As your interests and activities change, you may find yourself attracting new friends. Or, if all of your friends appear to be in the first category described above, you may want to purposefully go out and meet new friends. It is ideal to have friends who share the same values and lifestyle preferences. If you value health and a smoke-free environment, for example, you'll be most comfortable around non-smokers. If you are now very active, you'll enjoy friends who have a similar passion for sports, recreational activities, or the outdoors.

A great way to meet new friends is around shared activities. An athletic activity can help you maintain your weight loss and meet new friends. You can use the Internet to find a local running, hiking, or biking group. If there isn't one, start one. You can take dance classes or spinning classes and get to know people in the class.

You may find that you value your old friends but would like new friends for particular activities. There is nothing wrong with that. You can do different things with different friends. However, while much of your focus has been on weight loss, try not to make eating, body shape or weight, or exercise the main focus of your new friendships. You don't want to attract people who are obsessive and unhealthy in their pursuit of the perfect body or optimal fitness.

Remember that what you focus on expands. Thus, if you and your friends focus on discussing your growing waistline, it will probably expand. If you sit around talking about how miserable life is, you'll attract more misery into your life. If you obsess about every calorie you eat and become neurotic, you'll probably set yourself up for a backslide.

Select your friends by what they focus on. If potential friends focus on success and happiness, and you want those things and enjoy being around these people, spend more time with them. Your relationships can greatly support or hinder you in meeting your goals. Build those friendships that support you. Work on supporting others to guarantee all of your memberships in The Thin Club.

TIP

Create activity buddies. Replace food buddies with friends or dating partners who are active and share the same values and beliefs about being fit. Surrounding yourself with others who embody virtues you respect will help you (and them!) keep the weight off and increase your enjoyment of life post-weight-loss.

BEWARE THE FEEDER

You've probably come across some "feeders" on your road to weight loss. These are people who continue to enable unhealthy eating patterns and either unwittingly or knowingly sabotage your weight-loss process. Some feeders may get worse after you've lost the weight because they figure that you're thin now and they don't need to be as considerate as during the weight-loss phase. Other people feel that you're too thin now (even though you're a healthy weight; they were used to you eighty pounds bigger) and want to fatten you up a little to what they think looks good or healthy.

Larina suggests familiarizing yourself with the different types of feeders based on what motivates them to feed you. The types described below can apply to any form of relationship (not just intimate partners), including family members, significant others, and friends. Once you know what's driving them, you can understand how to best deal with them. Also think about whether any of these types of people describes you and your tendencies to feed others.

THE NURTURING FEEDER

This is the most benevolent and good-intentioned type of feeder. It's someone who truly wants to support your well-being but has many habits of her own to break. As you know, habits are difficult to change, so you should be able to empathize with the situation of the nurturing feeder.

Some people are taught from a young age that food means nurturing and protection from danger. They may have grown up without much food on the table in their family, so they feel it is very important to ensure that food is readily available for those they care about. Or they may have grown up in a family where food was equated with love: You feed people to show you love them and you eat the food prepared by other family members to express your gratitude and love. It is hard for them to separate food from love and security.

These feeders have good intentions and bad habits. They genuinely want to support you but are often unaware of their feeding behaviors. Or perhaps they realize that feeding is their way of nurturing but haven't learned any new behaviors. The best way to handle a nurturer is with nurturance. When you recognize that she is engaging in her feeding behavior, take a moment to thank her for her thoughtfulness. Then explain why food or the particular type of food she suggested is not in your best interest. Emphasize how much she'll *help* you by supporting your new healthy eating behaviors. Let her know other ways that she can nurture you, such as by going for walks with you or babysitting the kids while you go to the gym. Don't forget to thank her for all the nonfeeding-related nurturing actions.

THE JEALOUS FEEDER

The jealous feeder is often overweight himself. This is one of those "misery loves company" situations. The feeder figures that because he is overweight, you might as well be, too. This type of feeder may not even be aware of the jealousy that drives the feeding, but he is likely to be often envious of others' good fortunes and comparing himself to others. He may be competitive, judgmental, and pessimistic. He doesn't think that he (or you) can truly change.

Feeders who are driven by envy might have made your weight loss difficult by tempting you with tantalizing treats. As your self-esteem improved when you made healthy changes, his self-esteem plummeted. Rather than accepting his own responsibility for making positive changes in his life, he prefers to prove that it isn't just him who can't lose weight. So he (consciously or unconsciously) sabotages your weight loss to make himself feel better.

The jealous feeder can be difficult to deal with if you don't want to confront the jealousy head on. The best thing you can do is to use empathy to understand his situation and insecurities. You can compliment him for things that are not related to food or weight and encourage him to get involved in various activities to help build up his self-esteem. If these strategies don't work, you may need to remove yourself from eating-related activities when around him.

THE PASSIVE FEEDER

This type of feeder is one who, when told to jump, responds by saying "How high?" Being assertive and saying no is simply not in her repertoire of skills. She may realize that you don't truly want her to go on the ice cream run but feels powerless to stand up to your hormonally driven requests.

You may make this feeder uncomfortable by sending mixed messages. At one time you say that you want to have only healthy food in the house and then you're begging for some late-night pepperoni pizza. The problem with the passive feeder is that she is a true enabler of your overeating. The passive feeder may love you and it may pain her to see you pining for your favorite foods. She is probably someone who is uncomfortable with any conflict or negative emotion and would rather just give in to requests for food. This type of feeder is unlikely to barrage you with fattening foods. Instead, she finds it difficult to stand her ground when you make certain requests.

The best thing that you can do is to not put the passive feeder in a position of having to say no to you. Stop giving mixed messages about food so the passive feeder is able to be on the same page as you. You can let the passive feeder know how important and helpful it is when she *doesn't* feed you. If you happen to make the mistake of requesting the food you're trying not to eat, catch yourself and apologize. "I'm sorry. I know I asked you not to let me eat that and now I'm asking for it." When she is assertive and says no, thank her profusely to reinforce the assertiveness.

THE PEOPLE-PLEASING FEEDER

Everyone loves the receptionist who brings in fresh-baked chocolate chip cookies and the neighborhood socialite who hosts lavish parties with tons of delectable foods. Some people show their people-pleasing needs by feeding others. This is similar to the nurturing feeder, but different in some of the motives. People-pleasing feeders may get a specific social or personal benefit by being the providers of great food. They are sometimes people who are unsure of their worth as a person and try to keep interactions at a relatively superficial level ("Isn't this pie just divine?!"). They bask in the compliments from others and feel good when they feel needed.

The people-pleasing feeder has similar difficulties in saying no as the passive feeder experiences, but it often presents in a more subtle form. He can't be the one to bring the carrot and celery sticks because he would not be as appreciated as the one who brought triple-fudge brownies. Like the passive feeder, he has difficulty turning down requests for food because he has such a difficult time disappointing others.

To handle the people-pleasing feeder, show him that he is pleasing in ways that are not related to feeding you. For example, let him know how much you appreciate his friendly smile or cheerful attitude. If you cannot get the people-pleasing feeder to change, then decline eating with him. Do not allow yourself to be a pawn in his self-esteem. Recognize what is important to you and refuse to compromise your values to please others. Don't worry about disappointing him; he'll get over it. If you gave in and ate something just to please him by making him feel needed, you'll be the one to regret it and pay the consequences.

THE CONTROLLING FEEDER

The controlling feeder is similar to the jealous feeder but works in an even more malignant way. The jealous feeder is typically envious of your body as you slim down. The controlling feeder feels threatened by your new look because your weight loss might make you more attractive in the eyes of others. She feels that she cannot control you as well when you are thin and confident, and as a result she seeks to feed you to keep you submissive and in a position of less power in the relationship.

These types of persons can often escalate into becoming abusive. In fact, they may become more controlling as you shape your new body because they feel more vulnerable. If controlling you verbally doesn't work, they may resort to controlling you physically and threatening you. Not only can these behaviors sabotage your weight loss and lead to weight regain, they can be hurtful emotionally and physically. If you have children, it can place them in a dangerous situation.

Because the controlling feeder can be verbally, emotionally, or physically abusive, it is a good idea to receive some counseling or support to figure out how to handle the individual. You can call the National Domestic Violence Hotline (twenty-four hours a day, seven days a week) at 1-800-799-SAFE (7233) to get assistance or visit www.ndvh.org/help/help_in_area.html to find local support. Emotional abuse is as real and dangerous as physical abuse. Remember, damage to your self-esteem or confidence is part of emotional abuse.

THE SELF-ABSORBED FEEDER

The self-absorbed feeder is the husband who comes home with bags of cookies, chips, and candy even though he knows you're trying to keep the weight off. It is the wife who says, "If you don't want it, you don't have to eat it." It is your dining partner who knows that you are working to lose weight or keep off lost weight yet orders four rich, decadent courses when you go out for dinner.

These people can be seen as passive-aggressive because they often don't try to directly get you to eat, but they make it incredibly easy for you to slip back into bad habits. They don't consider how difficult weight maintenance may be for you or respect your wishes to not have particular foods around.

Sometimes you'll find that the self-absorbed feeder wants to get you to eat with her so she can have company when she eats the foods she wants. She may not like to eat alone, so she brings you in to help her feel better or enjoy her food. She may request that you prepare the meals that she wants or may refuse to go to restaurants with healthier options. She might be self-centered and judgmental—she wants to have her cake and eat it, too (pun intended). She thinks that you should be able to be fit and trim without any crimping of her lifestyle.

You will need to be assertive to come to a compromise with the self-absorbed feeder. Ideally, she sees how her behaviors negatively affect you and agrees to stop the sabotaging feeding. If she will not give up her favorite foods in the house or favorite restaurants, come to some compromises. For example, agree that because she wants ice cream sandwiches in the house and you do not, then you will occasionally have low-fat ice cream sandwiches in the house. Or make a list of restaurants where she can get her comfort food and you can get your confidence (healthy) food.

EATING-DISORDERED FEEDERS

People with eating disorders such as anorexia nervosa or bulimia nervosa are typically obsessed with food. Because of this, they enjoy preparing delicious foods for others. They like to watch others eat the food that they prepare. The reasons for this may be related to some of the feeder patterns we've discussed. Feeding others and resisting the food themselves can make anorexics feel like they have a lot of willpower and the ability to control food. Some do it to show others that they do not completely avoid food— they think that their being around food will alleviate others' concerns. Some eating-disordered patients get a vicarious sense of enjoyment by watching others eat. They are fascinated by what others eat, and feeding people gives them the opportunity to observe food being eaten.

If you are close to the eating-disordered feeder and he is not in treatment, then consider discussing some specific behaviors that he may want to address in treatment. Get help from a professional or a resource, such as www.something-fishy.org, to create a plan to best confront the individual you are concerned about. As with any of the feeder types, you can always remove yourself from the situation. You may need to be firm and keep repeating something like "Thanks, but I'm on my way out to get a big salad." These individuals may be fragile, so it's best to be firm and assertive without being harsh or demeaning.

TIP

Is there a feeder in your life? Is it you? Take some time to go through your relationships and think about whether anyone fits into these feeder patterns. Think about whether you may be serving as a feeder to someone else. Realize that some of the feeding behaviors are things that you may do for yourself to compensate for what you're not getting in a relationship. You may be, for example, acting as the nurturing feeder for yourself because your mate is not very nurturing. Most important, make a plan for change and commit to only healthy feeding relationships from now on!

THE OPPOSITE SEX FRIENDSHIP: WHAT'S THE DEAL?

It is a fact: Size matters when men are concerned. And I'm not talking about male anatomy, I'm talking about the female form. For the guys out there who wonder about women, most women I know would much rather look at a man without a beer belly.

In a world where everyone wants to be looked at as a total package—brains, accomplishments, and looks—being judged solely or initially on appearance can be daunting, even insulting. After all, appearance is hard to ignore—it's the first thing people see when they look at you. Take away the "looks factor" by adding enough weight to render yourself unattractive and "asexual," and you can only be judged by your intelligence, skills, and accomplishments.

Voilà! By blowing out our waistlines, we've created a platonic playing field! The problem is that while we might be taking our looks out of the picture, we are also crippling ourselves—not just in the world of guy-girl friendships but also in the overall universe, the work environment, the social scene, and just about every place in between. Appearance is very important and it does help us get ahead. And, yes, being perceived as charming, flirty, and fun by the opposite sex can actually bring benefits in the workplace and socially.

Flirting did not come naturally to me, and I never wanted to feel that a man liked me for my looks. And until I lost the weight, that was never a possibility. Male friends felt safe with me, and I with them. After the weight loss, the situation changed radically. For example, when I first lost the weight, my daughter would nudge me: "Mom, that guy is checking you out!" I would look at her incredulously.

"Get out! Why would he do that?"

" 'Cause you look hot," she exclaimed.

And soon enough, I began to notice the eyes, the subtle smiles, the flirting . . . and I was mortified. I didn't know where to look, what to do! As a former fatty, I had gone out of my way to avoid that kind of ridiculous behavior. "Don't women look stupid when they bat their eyes and act dumb or playful?" I thought. To me it made no sense. If you flirted you were sending a strong "I am interested!" signal.

And if you weren't interested, wasn't that misleading? Somehow, being heavy was so much less complicated! Who, other than an occasional oddball, would be interested in me for anything other than my brains? A male friend wanted my wisdom and my opinion, and that was all he needed from me.

I have come to appreciate the art of flirting—and yes, it is an art—and it largely comes from a feeling that I never had before, one of entitlement. Yes, I am an attractive woman, and when I converse with a nice man, I am entitled to enjoy his attention. It is part of my learning how to "take." And by giving a man attention in return, I am flattering him. But doesn't flirting lead to untoward behavior? As one of my informal "flirt coaches" explained to me, "Flirting with a man doesn't mean you're going to jump into bed with him. You don't have to act on every impulse, and if you choose to do that, well, that is totally within your control and should be a careful decision. But you can and should enjoy the attention a man gives you, knowing full well that you are an attractive, appealing woman who deserves to be showered with that flattery and adulation."

I guess the message hit home one day when I was driving on a major highway, feeling just a touch blue. I had had a rough week and a particularly difficult morning. I was en route to a business meeting and had dressed nicely. As I drove and sniffled a bit, I heard the sound of a diesel horn outside my window. I briefly glanced and saw a garbage truck in the right-hand lane. Out popped a hand—a male hand—and as the horn blared again, the hand gave me the "thumbs up" sign. I smiled and accepted the compliment gladly. It made my day!

Peter, a divorced man who underwent not only bariatric surgery for weight loss but also an extensive operation to remove the loose skin left over from years of excess fat, said he was flattered but initially completely unnerved by the attention he seemed to suddenly be getting from women. Women who used to be "just friends" seemed to be giving him more than friendly vibes, the kind that would make him wonder exactly what they meant when they would help him arrange carpools and then stick around his house to talk for hours on end. Even the married ones, he said, seemed to be giving off different vibes. Was it some kind of new cologne, his new sleek body, or his newfound confidence in his appearance? Perhaps it was a combination of factors, but Peter had to learn how to respectfully deflect certain overtures that he felt were inappropriate, and to sit back and enjoy the ones that were merely appreciative. "Just because a woman appreciates me, it doesn't mean I have to run for the hills or even necessarily do something about it," he explained. "Sometimes a good conversation is just a satisfying conversation."

A friend of the opposite sex can provide the best ego boost someone could ever ask for. Will being thin make it more difficult to maintain nonsexual friendships with others? The simple answer is, it may but it doesn't have to. There is nothing wrong with a male-female friendship in which two people are respectful, attractive, and attentive yet don't feel the passionate need to jump into bed with one another. A friendship or a neighborly or work relationship with someone of the opposite sex can be an illuminating and healthy experience, in spite of—or perhaps because of—the fact that you are looking and feeling your very best.

MEMBER SUPPORT

Ongoing support is one of the most important factors in your continuous success with weight management. There are tons of ways to get support. The most obvious is through your own social networks, including friends and family. While these support systems are wonderful and important, not everyone has them, and even if you do, you want to use them wisely. It is sometimes a better idea to rely on professional networks for support so that you get the right information and type of support and so that you don't overuse your personal networks.

THE POWER OF SUPPORT GROUPS

Support groups can be very helpful because you are around people who face similar issues, stresses, fears, struggles, joys, celebrations, and ideas. If you are already in The Thin Club, it is better to join a support group with people who have also already lost the weight rather than a group with people who are working to lose weight. If you can't find one around you, begin one.

Many people find support groups run by organizations such as Weight Watchers to be helpful. Remember that people around you will help you to shape your own reality, so surround yourself with people who are doing what you want to do. If the "support" group is mostly a "bitch session" about how horrible it is to restrict portion sizes and give up fried food, it is less likely to help you. Support groups work best when they not only give you a place to vent but also provide inspiration and encouragement for meeting your goals. So, while you can empathize with each other about how difficult it is to eat only half a slice of bread with dinner, be sure to also discuss how great your energy level is now and why the change is worth it.

Support groups also work best when a professional or trained peer is present as a facilitator. You don't want to rely on misinformation from other group members. Sometimes when Larina hears people who have been successful with weight loss sharing their tips with others and telling them "You *have to* try this!" she wishes that they wouldn't. What works for one person is not necessarily what works for others, and there are some universal principles, proven in clinical research, that are important to uphold. Larina cautions people: What works for you is exactly that—what works for *you.* Some people do very well with portion control and can regularly eat all their favorite foods. Others have great difficulty with sugary foods and need to keep them off limits. Remember that The Thin Club members entered the club by way of different weight-loss strategies. And what works for losing weight and what works for keeping it off are often different. Be careful about recommending specific actions to others because they may not work for them and may even work against them.

TIP

Make sure your support is supportive. Don't select groups of people who complain and focus on the problems. Instead, select groups that are positive and inspiring for you. Use the groups to exchange great tips, success stories, recipes, and experiences. If you can't find a great support group, start one yourself. You can span geography by using a teleconference format if you live in a rural area or think your group could benefit by geographic diversity.

PSYCHOTHERAPY FOR DEEPER ISSUES

Individual therapy is a powerful vehicle that can help you break maladaptive patterns and manners of responding to situations. For example, therapy can help you if you have an abusive or neglectful past. If you have symptoms of posttraumatic stress disorder, like nightmares, vivid memories, or physical symptoms like heart racing and sweating, or if you avoid situations that may remind you of the trauma, seek a psychological evaluation. There are highly effective forms of cognitive-behavioral therapy for this and other anxiety disorders. For more information or to find a therapist, see the Notes section for referral information.

Therapy can also help you with things like:

- Improving your self-esteem, body image, and self-concept
- Reducing depression or the likelihood of a relapse of depression
- Managing anger and an explosive temperament
- Reducing stress or improving your use of time
- Adjusting to major life changes
- Leaving or managing an abusive relationship

WEIGHT-LOSS COACHING

You've probably heard about life coaching or weight-loss coaching because the field of coaching has become very popular and has received a great deal of media attention. As a weight-loss coach and a psychologist, Larina hears people frequently ask about the difference between coaching and therapy. They are actually quite different. While *therapy* aims to help you overcome a troubled past, maladaptive thoughts and behavioral patterns, things that are greatly interfering with your life or functioning, and deep-seated issues, *coaching* focuses on the present and helps you reach your highest goals in a strengths- and solution-based approach for healthy people with ambition and motivation.

Some clients pursue coaching and therapy simultaneously. Some complete therapy and then move on to coaching. Coaching by itself is not appropriate for clients who would be best helped by dealing with clinical issues, such as a history of abuse or serious depression. On the other hand, some clients do not need therapy because they don't have clinical issues, but they could benefit significantly from coaching.

One area that therapy and coaching share is education. Both therapists and coaches provide clients with resources and information. Coaching reflects an equal relationship or partnership between client and coach. The coach supports the client by holding the client accountable and helping her achieve her vision. Coaching is often beneficial in the maintenance phase of weight loss to keep a client on track and help create new goals (about physical fitness or other aspects of life) and achieve them.

Larina has found that several of her coaching clients successfully lose their weight and then pursue other dreams through coaching. It's a great time to expand your successful mindset and bring happiness and achievement to other areas of your life. For example, several of her clients began businesses they'd always dreamed of having after they'd achieved significant weight loss. Another client, newly confident, decided to pursue a new line of work. Many people gain momentum to promote themselves and forge ahead in their careers. Other clients seek to create balanced lifestyles, reduce stress, and enjoy more time with friends and families. Improving relationship communication or seeking out new relationships are other common goals of coaching.

Remember that success breeds more success, and the happier and more fulfilled you are as a whole person, the more likely you are to stay in The Thin Club. You'll have the energy and drive to eat healthy and exercise and pursue other hopes and dreams. If you are interested in coaching, interview some coaches to see who may be a good fit for you. Coaching is not currently a licensed profession, so be sure that your coach has credentials and testimonials from past clients. Many coaches possess certifications from their coach training school or the International Coach Federation (ICF).

TIP

Not sure if therapy or coaching is more appropriate for you? Seek the counsel of a professional. If you have a feeling that therapy could help you, get an evaluation with a psychologist and let him or her know that you'd like a treatment recommendation at the end of the evaluation. You could also complete an initial session with a coach to get another perspective. Many coaches give free initial sessions or consultations so you could use that time to address the question of whether therapy or coaching seems more appropriate.

There are now many coaches who are also mental health professionals (with master's or doctorate degrees in psychology, social work, or counseling). Coaches with these qualifications would be your best bet in answering the question of whether to pursue coaching and/or therapy. If you and the professional decide it would be a good idea to do both simultaneously, do not do therapy with your coach—keep them separate. Your coach could help you get a referral to a psychologist or vice versa.

SOUL FOOD

Feeding the Spirit

"I'M LOSING WEIGHT," MY FRIEND CONFIDED IN ME happily. "I have to, so I can allow myself to eat a big slice of cheesecake on the holiday." The Jewish holiday of Shavuot, a celebration of the Jews' receiving the oral and written traditions and bringing the first fruits to the Temple, traditionally includes at least one dairy meal. Among the traditions, which include staying up all night to learn the holy texts and listening to the Ten Commandments as they are read in synagogue, is the custom of eating cheesecake to commemorate certain dietary laws that were handed down on that day. I couldn't help but wonder how the message got so garbled, with my friend perceiving Shavuot as "The Cheesecake Holiday" for which she must carve out a calorie allowance ahead of time.

The Jewish holidays are usually full of food. I was raised Orthodox, and food was perceived as spiritual sustenance, as well as a communal experience. Over the years, the lines blurred and were translated into indulging in some of the fattiest, greasiest, carb-ridden foods ever (potato latkes, noodle kugel, jelly donuts, bagels, cheesecake, hamantaschen, rugelach, and the most decadent cakes to celebrate every *simcha* (happiness) or holiday.

Even weddings are frequently centered more on food and less on the occasion, the dancing, and the speeches. Many weddings feature copious amounts of precisely the kind of food that packs on the pounds. One recent wedding I attended, held at 6 P.M. on a weeknight, offered tables full of cakes oozing frosting and filling in lieu of a cocktail hour. While some of the guests seemed bewildered by the array of desserts put in front of them in what appeared to be the wrong order, others were digging into mousse cakes and caramel éclairs. By the time the bride and groom walked down the aisle, many of the guests were nodding off as their sugar highs wore off. The beautiful religious aspects of the religious ceremony got literally swallowed up in the frenzy to feast.

Is this the way God meant food to be enjoyed? Interestingly, while the texts indicate the importance of celebrating happiness, Jewish philosophers and sages have never advocated "pigging out." Quite the contrary, Jews—and many other religious groups—are encouraged to be controlled in what they eat, when they eat, and how they eat. For me, the spiritual connection has been a key one—the spiritual "third" angle of the Body, Mind, and Spirit triangle—and one that has given me solace, comfort, and strength when I have felt that nothing else was in my control.

Blessings are chanted before drinking and eating, and grace is recited afterward. In the appropriate religious light, food is always viewed as a gift from God, one that is continually provided especially to the faithful to fuel our spiritual being and refresh our soul. As I lost weight, I discovered the power of prayer. Each Saturday found me at the synagogue asking for much-needed help—trying to connect to God, recharge my battery, refresh my soul, and get the tools that I needed to fuel my weight loss. Eventually, I set aside time each day to pray. I prayed for strength, I prayed for perspective, I prayed for energy. And in praying I found energy similar to the energy I feel after I've exercised, as well as relaxation similar to the state I achieve in hypnosis.

RELIGION AND FOOD: A BUILT-IN CONTROL MECHANISM

The attitude of daily and constant attention to what and why we consume the foods that we do, plus the recognition that we don't have to hoard or overeat in order to feed our collective body, mind, or spirit, certainly enhance any diet plan. Indeed, some control over food is built into most structured religions. In fact, many religions have fasts as well as feasts—days, sometimes even months of ritual deprivation of certain foods, or in the case of some religions, all food. Lent, Ramadan, meatless Fridays, Yom Kippur, Tisha BaAv—the object lesson being that our lives need not center on food and, in fact, doing without food can be spiritually as well as physically enlightening. Food intake is to be controlled and balanced in order to preserve our spiritual nature.

In dieting as in religion, I found similar resistance to setting aside time and keeping myself tied to a schedule. Braving the elements and getting myself to the synagogue is not always easy, and focusing hard on the prayers and sermons can be challenging, yet like exercise, when I manage to do it I always feel stronger afterwards for having done so.

"God is the ultimate safety net," says former stunt-woman Desiree Ayres, now a pastor at In His Presence

Church in the Warner Center, Woodland Hills, California, near Hollywood. Desiree relied on her spiritual connection to be healed of anorexia, bulimia, and compulsive binge eating, and she has written *God Hunger,* an inspirational guide to breaking addictions, particularly food-related ones.

"Healing and faith are so intertwined," explains Desiree. "Turning to God and trusting in His ultimate wisdom and guidance allows you to address addictions and celebrate your body image as a gift from God that must be cherished." The church, which Ayres co-pastors with her husband, Mel, a former actor, now Senior Pastor, is housed in a 40,000-square-foot, 1,100-seat building. Weekly attendance is typically over 1,500, including many Hollywood professionals—everyone from camera grips to casting agents.

Her book details Desiree's battles with weight and body image. "Admitting that I had a problem was the hardest thing to do," recalls Desiree. "It was a cataclysmic revelation that set me on the road to recovery." Her first step in healing was to confide in her husband, who counseled her and encouraged her to pray and turn to God. As Desiree delved into the Bible, prayer, and spiritual studies, she gradually found the strength to deal with the problems that were causing her to overeat and feel empty inside.

"I replaced food as a comfort source," she explains. "When you immerse yourself in the spiritual aspect of life, you don't have to fill yourself with food." Eventually, Desiree began to recognize a similar void in others, and people with weight issues began seeking her spiritual solace. Here are some of Desireé's *God Hunger* tips:

1. Start each day with a spiritual breakfast! Read the Bible for ten minutes when you first wake up and ask God to speak to you. Follow it with a healthy breakfast! Prayer plus food will speed your metabolism.

2. Make all your food "soul food." Before you put food in your mouth, ask God, "Is this good for the body that you created in your image and likeness?" Listen to your inner voice, and if the answer is no, resist your impulse to indulge or overindulge.

3. Visualize anyone who has done you wrong, and forgive them. This eliminates "victim mentality" and helps you make room in your life for better thoughts and feelings.

IN GOD WE TRUST—NO NEED TO HOARD

From its very beginning, the Bible is chock-full of references to food. The Garden of Eden was brimming with food, and Adam and Eve enjoyed it until Eve took the one thing that was not on the divine diet. Food as sacrifice followed: food used as gifts from man to man, and man to God. Bounty was a gift God gave to His faithful. And those who recognized their sustenance as Godly gifts had a sense of satisfaction, even if they didn't have quite as much as their neighbor in the tent down the way. Food throughout the Bible is integral and never is to be taken for granted. From the story of Cain and Abel, to Esau and Jacob's lentil exchange over the birthright, to Joseph's being named Viceroy to the Pharaoh and manager of the silos, food and faith go hand in hand.

Manna, the food that fell from heaven to sustain the Jews during their desert journey, fell in the precise amounts that each person needed—no more and no less. Just prior to the Sabbath, the desert clan was allowed to collect a double portion that lasted them through the day of rest. On any day other than the Sabbath, if anyone tried to take extra portions—to hoard the manna—they were amazed to find that portion spoiled. The message here was if one trusts in God, there is no need to hoard or feel deprived, even though Jews who keep the kosher laws are certainly limited in what they are allowed to eat—no pork, shellfish, and only animals that are slaughtered ritually. They are encouraged to take their fill, keep their eyes on their own plates, and know that God provides exactly what is needed to sustain and enable them to serve God.

TIP

Try prayer on the run. If setting aside specific time for prayer is hard, combine it with your exercise routine. Prayers can be uttered as you run or walk and enjoy the nature of God's beauty. Roaming the Judean hills and exploring caves and streams in and around Jerusalem inspired King David. If you aren't able to pen your own prayer, download some prayers, sermons, or religious songs on your iPod. It will boost your workout and make you feel spiritual and fit!

My mother, who is very religious, had been extremely overweight when I was young and used to smoke a lot. Her doctor had prescribed diet pills. One day he told her that he could no longer provide her with the pills she so depended on. So my mother turned to prayer. She found that by saying prayers before and after meals, she created a sort of control mechanism. If she didn't want to say a lengthy Grace, she wouldn't indulge in certain foods. Praying in some way satisfied her oral fixation. By mouthing words to God, she was able to resist the persistent cravings that hounded her. She lost weight and stopped smoking. The power of prayer is wonderful.

TIP

Say amazing grace. Bracket your food prayers so that you thank God before and after you eat (snacks as well as meals). It will slow down your eating, help you appreciate the significance of the bounty you are about to or have just received, and will help you feel that you and God are a partnership in your nutrition and weight loss.

Born in A.D. 1135, Rabbi Moses ben Maimon, also known as Maimonides, was a Jewish physician and healer and the author of many texts, both medical and philosophical. His credo of moderation—advising people to always leave some food on their plates and to eat to live, not live to eat—was truly ahead of its time. Groups like Overeaters Anonymous, based on twelve-step methodology, incorporate the recognition of a higher power in their efforts to control behavior. By understanding what is in our control, and what may not be, we achieve a sense of balance.

TIP

Set a time each day or week. Just as you do for exercise, set a specific time to pray or meditate. You can begin with once a week, but don't miss a session! Add on daily prayers and watch your concentration and focus improve!

One of Larina's clients told her that she was able to use her relationship with God to help motivate her to achieve her weight loss and improve her body image. She used prayer to center and ground her. Prayer helped her to gain strength, calm her mind when she was stressed (and for her, stress often led to eating), and resist temptations. She had a difficult time with her body image—seeing herself as "fat and ugly" even after she began to lose weight. But she reminded herself that she was beautiful in God's eyes—fat, thin, or in between. She was able to focus on her inner beauty and on being a good person and accepted herself for who she was. By improving her body image through seeing herself as God sees her, she improved her self-esteem and increased her ability to keep weight off.

TIP

Pen your own prayer. When you can't find an appropriate prayer, create your own. If you weren't raised religious or aren't quite sure how to pray, it's easy. Begin by acknowledging that you are seeking help, then cite your request(s). Conclude by promising to look beyond your own small universe and to give back to those less fortunate than yourself. By putting your own situation in perspective, you are not only helping others but also helping yourself!

MAKING UP FOR LOST TIME

Reclaiming Yourself

"YOU *ARE* THE FORTY-YEAR-OLD VIRGIN!" MY FRIEND David exclaimed as his eyes went back and forth from the "fat" photo to the now-thin me. "There's so much you haven't done! Do you realize you have to start living for the first time now?" And he was right. Living an over-weight or obese childhood, adolescence, early adulthood, or adulthood can lead to the feeling that you have missed out on important developmental milestones. I had never tried on a prom dress. I had never finessed my flirting, en-joyed shaking my booty (it was too big!), or sat in a bar. I never got to walk down Fifth Avenue wearing trendy fash-ions and feeling that they fit my figure and personality. I never played the debutante or leading role. I was always the fat, brainy buddy!

So now it is my time to shine! But how do I "shine" and still be "appropriate"? Or do I have to be appropriate? Should I write off the years I've missed and just relax into middle age—or somehow try to get them back? While some people have a midlife crisis, I had a "missed-life cri-sis." I spent most of my twenties dressed in ugly muumuus and elastic waistband suits. I never had the energy to play and run in the yard with my children. Why hadn't I gone paintball shooting or rock climbing with my son when he was a teenager? Because I was too busy baking, cooking, or eating. I'd never tried hiking, biking, or skiing, either. It felt like I'd missed out on a lifetime—a lifetime marked by inertia, by deliberately taking myself out of certain joyful experiences, like swinging on a porch swing or scuba diving. I just couldn't participate, afraid that my weight would break the wooden swing.

Now that I've lost the weight, I feel as if I've walked into a movie at the middle. I've missed the first part of life and there is no rewind! There is a certain sadness in knowing that I can never ever get those years back. And there is that ever-present desire to somehow recapture some of the missed moments. So I made a list of Old Me and New Me, to understand what I missed and what I have reclaimed. And here is what my list looks like. If you are going through this process, make your own list—if nothing else, it will show you just how far you've come.

OLD ME	NEW ME
Avoided parties at all costs.	Is learning to like them, one party at a time.
Would wear shirts over my bathing suit.	Bought my first bikini and wore it with pride.
Always wore my shirt out.	Always tuck in, wear clingy clothes.
Would avoid strenuous exercise.	Love the feeling of sweat connecting with my body.
Hated undressing in locker rooms.	Posed for a semi-nude photo shoot for book.

OLD ME	NEW ME
Thought flirting was demeaning.	Have become successful at flirting and use it to my advantage.
Took sedentary vacations.	Take action-filled vacations— rappelling, flying plane, etc.
Wore dark colors.	Love to bling it up in bright, eye-popping colors.
Limited sexual positioning.	The sky is the limit!
Would never even try for the best-looking guy in the room.	I look. I like. I go for it!

HOT! NOW WHAT?

One friend who is halfway to her weight-loss goal has taken up activities she has always wanted to try, like flying a plane and riding a motorcycle. She is going on adventure vacations and taking more time away from the kids. These were things she had back-burnered for years while she lived for everyone else, losing years. Her metamorphosis was triggered by the death of her father and by health problems caused by her obesity. She took control and committed herself to a slow but steady weight loss and an ongoing exercise routine. Her entire outlook shifted.

"I realized that life is too short," she told me. "And if I continued my patterns it would be even shorter. There was so much I still wanted to do. Now I can do everything I had always wanted to do—and even some things I didn't imagine I could ever do."

OK, so now that you're svelte, is it time to rekindle some of the old you? Can you relive some of the times you may have "missed" because you were overweight and unable or uncomfortable dressing, acting, or interacting in certain ways? And now that you look good and you're getting those affirming looks, do you find yourself shamelessly giggling and batting your eyelashes at the most inappropriate times (like at Uncle Henry's funeral)?

These are all questions that you're probably asking yourself now that you have the rest of your life in front of you in a thin body. But you can't forget the past and all those things you never did. It can be healthy to reclaim a lost past. Larina cautions, however, that it is unhealthy to live in the past. The question "Now what?" is an important one to answer. We'll help you create a plan for reclaiming your past in the here and now. But first, let's consider how the weight loss might have affected you and your reflections on the past.

MIXED FEELINGS

Many people describe significant weight loss as an entirely new chapter or new beginning, especially if they have been overweight most of their lives. The longer you were overweight, the more likely it is that the weight loss will bring up sentimental thoughts about your life as a heavy person. Expect your emotions to run the gamut from extreme happiness and gratitude for where you are now to sadness and mourning about where you've been.

Thinking through the things that you missed out on over the years can be very upsetting. Some people experience grief for the life they lost being hostage to fat and food. One of Larina's clients once told her about losing weight, "I'm having a hard time forgiving myself for not doing this earlier. I feel like I lost out on twenty years of life and it's all my fault."

Many people have thoughts like this one. They wish they could relive those moments. They feel sad for the "fat kid" that used to be teased mercilessly by his classmates. They want to comfort the heavy teenager who, too embarrassed to eat in front of others, sneaks her food into the bathroom or waits until she gets home to voraciously eat. They wish they would have gone to prom, had the courage to ask people out on dates, shopped in the trendy stores, presented themselves confidently in the workplace, gone outside to play sports with their kids, or, perhaps most important, felt good about themselves when they had a glimpse of their reflection in glass while walking down the street, instead of feeling mortified and humiliated. All these memories can be hard to deal with, but it's important to work through them and feel good about where you are now.

TIP

Remind yourself that all emotions about your past are normal. Don't try to fight off the emotions that come up when you think through the lost time. Accept your feelings—the good, the bad, and the ugly.

It sounds strange, but part of you might miss your formerly fat self. You may long for the times when you were able to enjoy food with wild abandon. You may miss the feeling of eating vast quantities of food and eating until you felt stuffed. You might wish you could still eat whatever you want without considering calories and how much exercise you need to do to burn them off.

The other emotion that you are likely to experience is fear. When you think through your past and the hardships and difficulties you experienced because of your weight, there's an intense fear about "What if this new body isn't here to stay and I have to go through that all over again?" If you have been on the yo-yo diet track and have seen your weight go up and down, you probably have experienced this feeling that the new you is too good to be true and that it's unlikely to last.

TIP

Embrace the fat past. If you find yourself feeling down or nervous when you think through the difficulties of living life as an overweight person, flip the coin over and think about the positive things that resulted from the struggles. There's research that people who have experienced a trauma or a major loss in life end up not only surviving but also thriving when they think of the positive aspects of the difficult event. Work to create meaning for yourself about why you went through what you went through. Try not to regret it, but embrace it.

It may be that you wouldn't have developed important nonphysical aspects of yourself had you not had the experiences you had. Maybe you're now more empathic, loving, nurturing, or strong for what you've been through. Take a few moments to write down the meaning that you can take away from the struggles in your fat past.

RECLAIMING YOURSELF THROUGH "THE NEW YOU"

The question to ask yourself now is, "Is the aspect of my lost past that I missed out on still important to me?" And if so, the next question is, "Is there a way that I can tailor the experience to the life I'm living now?" Let's say, for example, that you had a pretty dismal dating life when you were in college. While your cohorts got dolled up in their cocktail dresses for semiformal mixers, you sat home with a big bowl of popcorn and a bag of cookies. Even if you felt comfortable going to a semiformal, you couldn't find a cute dress in your size. Now you're ready to go shopping and accept more cocktail party invitations. Or perhaps even throw one yourself!

First, think about what part of that experience is important to you today. Is it looking nice in a flattering dress? Is it being admired by other women? Is it having the hottest guy at the party notice you from across the room? Once you have an idea of the part of the lost time that you long for, ask yourself, "Why?" The answer to this question will help you figure out how to make up for lost time.

TIP

List the lost past. Write down all the important things you feel you missed out on before you lost the weight. Then think about why. Put your list in order of importance for what matters to you most now. You may find that when you were eighteen, not being asked to the prom was the biggest deal in the world, but now you could care less. Once you know what is important to you today, it's time to start planning how to do those things.

Now, think about whether it is appropriate, beneficial, and possible to incorporate the lost situation into your current life. If you missed out on flirting with cute fraternity boys back in college, you can't exactly relive that moment, especially if you're now married with kids. But you can dress up in a flattering outfit and have a romantic evening with your husband.

TIP

Make it work for you now. Think about how you can re-create a lost moment so it enhances the life you're living right now. (Proceed with caution when you reclaim the past because you're not living in the past, you're living in the present.)

When you plan how to reclaim your past, you may want to get a trusted friend or family member to serve as a reality check. This can help you learn to not live in the past and to act appropriately. For this to work, you need to vow to be open and appreciative when the friend gives you feedback. If, for example, your sister sees you heading out to a parent-teacher conference in the Daisy Duke shorts you had always wanted to wear, she can suggest another option, and you can consider which outfit is the best choice for the situation (and, of course, thank her for the input).

"You should try skydiving sometime," my colleague said excitedly. He was an experienced skydiver. Actually, it was something I had thought about years ago, but never bothered to do because of my weight. "Next Sunday?" He looked at me expectantly. I yearned to say, "Sure," but thought twice, considering the heart problems I had in the past. Maybe it wouldn't be such a great idea. While jumping out of planes was something I always had dreamed about, I knew on some level that, at this point and time, the window of opportunity had closed. I thought long and hard, and instead booked a lesson with a local flight school. I went up in a Cessna with a flight instructor who taught me a bit about flying and let me take the wheel (known as the yoke), which did not at all imperil my health and gave me a thrill nonetheless. It was a cool compromise and something I wouldn't have done while I was heavy. It was a perfectly acceptable and appropriate solution.

Whatever way you decide to reclaim your past, the most important thing is to vow never again to miss out on anything that is important to you because of food or weight. Plan to *carpe diem*—live each moment to its fullest, even those challenging holiday parties.

ELEVEN

SHOPPING

Dressing the New You

I SAT ACROSS FROM THE MARKETING DIRECTOR AT the meeting and felt his eyes on me. He was staring at the see-through lacy top with black sports bra peeking from underneath, framed by my size 8 Dolce & Gabbana pants suit jacket. What was wrong with showing off my hot bod? I was proud of my new figure—maybe a little *too* proud, judging by the smirk that played across this man's face at this particular business meeting. He didn't seem to be listening to my expert strategy advice; he was too busy staring directly at my chest! The president of the company (also male) exchanged glances with him and they smiled ever so slightly, eyebrows raised, at each other. Was it getting hot in that room or what? Should I be enjoying this attention-getting moment or unfurl the nearest legal folder to cover up my peekaboo top? It was a fashion faux pas I was not likely to forget anytime soon.

Just because you can wear something, doesn't mean you *should* wear it. And what works for one occasion may be scandalous for another. That goes for dressing when you're heavy, as well as when you have joined The Thin Club. But after shopping for years at Lane Bryant, and then being thrust into the world of couture and runway fashion, your barometer and judgment may be a bit off from the sheer excitement of believing that you can actually look sexy and alluring, and downright fabulous, in beautiful clothing.

Shopping can become an obscene smorgasbord. Just as my former self used to indulge in eating fests that sometimes took me miles out of my way to exotic pie shops and the greasiest burger joints with the saltiest french fries, now I sometimes find myself looking for the most décolleté blouse on the rack, without considering the fact that it is probably an item that won't (or shouldn't) get much wear in my day-to-day life. And just as I've learned to develop the "You don't *need* it!" sense when I'm craving french fries, I have had to develop that same sensibility while combing through the racks at Century 21.

TIP

Shop for quality not quantity. Look for some wardrobe items that you will be able to wear for a long time. You will have some beautiful pieces that you really feel good in and you will not need to build a new wing on your house for closet space.

I have learned that even though my careful attention to diet and exercise has earned me "the right to dress tight," dressing tight is not always the appropriate way to go. How do you develop a fashion sense and judgment after years of wearing elastic waistbands?

FEAR FACTOR: WHY SHOPPING CAN BE SCARY

Shopping is hardly a problem, my already thin friends told me. Shopping is supposed to be *fun*! And my friends who hadn't yet joined The Thin Club scoffed in envy at the fact that I viewed shopping as something of a challenge: "What a Drama Queen! Complaining about having to go out and buy herself smaller clothes for her new body! Hmmph!"

Before I resolved to finally lose weight and the weight loss had begun, I had given up dressing nicely. I never knew what would look good, so why bother? As long as it fit (and elastic waists were a must back then), I wore it, with big, baggy jackets designed to hide my big, baggy body. Shopping was an experience I dreaded. Trudging through "fat departments," facing the dressing-room mirror, getting "the look" when I timidly ventured into the "regular" boutiques, dealing with salespeople who made it clear that I didn't belong in *their* store—it all translated into sheer stress, even when I was a size that could be found in the boutique.

Even when you are finally thin, the memories don't fade easily. While we were still heavy, some of us may have ventured into trendy boutiques with European sizes (36, 38, 39) that meant nothing to us, until we hopelessly tried to squish into them. Still others may have suffered humiliation when they were rebuffed at stores that seldom stock anything in excess of a size 10. So here we are, ready to venture back into the lion's den with our new size 6 bodies. Is it any wonder that you sweat and experience heart palpitations before you even open the door of that boutique? When the salesperson glides over to you, you wonder if she's going to sneer at you or help you.

When I first began shopping, the name of the game was "hide my belly"; as I began losing weight, other body parts that needed camouflage caught my eye. But after several weeks of staying "on program," clothes began fitting just a bit better—then looser—and eventually the skirt that hadn't been worn in a season went from being a bit snug to a drapey hip-hugger. That is when the "big reveal" happened for me. As my clothes drooped, friends and colleagues began to notice and voilà, it became unavoidable: time for a whole new shopping trip.

Yet for me, who hadn't seen the inside of a non-plus-sized department in a while, there were attitude adjustments to make before I could comfortably hit the sale circuit at Lord & Taylor. And I was clueless about where to start. What size was I? Who knew? Even the sizes had changed since I'd last worn "normal" (a.k.a. non-plus-size) clothing. The sizes had gotten bigger; they weren't the way I'd remembered them. I stood on the sales floor and wondered where to start.

As I lost weight, even underwear became a mystery. I used to think that Victoria indeed had a secret, namely that she hated fat people. The first time I ventured into a Victoria's Secret store post-weight-loss, I felt like Alice in Wonderland fallen down the rabbit hole. I had gone from a 42D bra to a "who knows" what size, and while I had never in my life considered buying a thong or something else sexy, now the notion didn't seem quite as bizarre. I still had reservations, but I didn't have a clue as to how or what to buy. When I finally got up the nerve to approach a saleswoman, she asked me what size I was. When I told her I didn't know, she looked at me like I was nuts.

My solution was to whip out my "fat pictures" and show her why I couldn't help her figure out my figure. Instant sympathy and admiration! She immediately helped me find a bra that fit the new me to a tee, and another that pushed things up and filled them out, and another, and another—well, you get the picture. I never knew there were so many choices and so many styles.

My confusion didn't end in the underwear department. The styles that I bought to be "slenderizing"—ugh . . . my mother's word, a euphemism for "It makes even *you*, a baby elephant, look halfway decent, even though you aren't thin like your cousin!"—when I was a size 16 were no longer flattering when I was a size 10. And as I made my way down to even smaller sizes, I knew I no longer had to follow the old "no horizontal stripes," "black hides figure flaws" rules, but I had no idea what rules to follow now that I no longer had a belly or hips to hide.

I saw designer names that I had heard of somewhere but had never seen up close before. As I perused the racks, my eyes automatically led me to clothing that was way too big for me! And while lots of clothes fit, not everything made me look good. My first post-weight-loss shopping spree yielded a halter top that I spilled out of, a pair of Versace turquoise jeans that hugged me so tight that my belly hung over the top, and three T-shirts that I swore were my size but were hanging on me when I tried them on.

TIP

When you go shopping, bring a picture of your previous self as well as a current picture. Use them to show yourself the difference. Use them to enthusiastically tell the sales clerk about your weight loss and enlist his or her help in finding your current size.

There are a lot of factors involved in shopping. Picking out, purchasing, and wearing clothes, according to Larina, is a complex psychological and behavioral process. This is especially true for people who are currently overweight or who were overweight and are now members of The Thin Club. She adds that choosing what to buy and wear involves deciding how much you are worth spending on, thinking about what is flattering or the most concealing of perceived flaws, knowing what really does look good on you, picturing yourself looking nice in the new outfit—this list could go on and on.

TIP

If you've lost a lot of weight, this one can have you trying on a lot of clothes, but it is very effective. Go to a store and get an outfit in the size that you used to wear. Then get the same outfit in every size between that size and your current size. So, if you used to be a 16 and do not know what you are now, get 16 down to 6 and try them all on. If the store does not carry the size that you used to be, get the largest item that store does carry or bring one of your previous outfits in with you. This exercise will help you to see your current size and can also aid you in creating a more accurate body image of yourself following weight loss.

DRESSING A NEW BODY

When people lose weight, the act of getting dressed becomes so challenging because of four primary factors:

body-image distortions, lack of shopping confidence, fear, and wanting it all.

DISTORTIONS OF BODY IMAGE

Larina recalls that, one day when she was shopping for a winter jacket, she tried on a huge, black down jacket that made her look like a bowling ball with a fluffy furry collar. As a naturally petite person, she was able to discount the big image she saw in front of her in the mirror. The image in the mirror and the image in her mind did not go together. But Larina has much more experience with the body image in her mind, since she has been carrying it around for some time. She selected the image of the small person (who happens to be wearing a big jacket) and moved on. She told herself, "That doesn't look good, but something else will."

Now, let's say that you are a recent entrant into The Thin Club and are looking at yourself in the mirror—a new svelte woman looks back at you from the mirror. As someone who had developed an image of an overweight person, your body image may no longer match the image in the mirror. Since body image forms over time and does not automatically adjust when you lose weight, Larina says it's not uncommon for your image to still be one of the heavy person. The image in the mirror and the image in your mind do not match, so you go with the image in your mind: you as an overweight person.

So, what happens next? Confusion. You do not know what sizes to try on because the image tells you that you are overweight. You do not know what is flattering because the typical thought is, "Nothing is flattering—just get what best hides you." You may go to the other extreme and wear something that is way too small simply because you do not know what fits.

The negative body image that can persist after weight loss can have a significant impact on your shopping experiences and on your ability to keep the weight off. According to a recent study, those who retain a negative body image have more struggles to keep weight off. So putting on a new outfit and being able to say "I look fabulous" can help you keep the weight off. It can also help you realign your body image with your new thinner appearance.

One way to be able to say "I look fabulous" is to change the appearance assumptions that you may hold, such as the idea that appearance is one of the important elements of life or that your life would only be better if you changed your look. Research shows that if you hold certain assumptions about the critical importance of appearance in your life, you are more likely to have a negative body image. Larina cites a study that shows that 73 percent of people who held appearance assumptions had body dissatisfaction, whereas only 14 percent of those who did not hold these assumptions had body dissatisfaction.

Body image is more complex than good versus bad and usually falls within a continuum. Gannett Health Services at Cornell University created a model showing the spectrum of body image and the impacts on eating and confidence. The abbreviated version is below.

Flexible, healthy eating and confidence
about body size and shape

Preoccupied with food and dieting
and attempt to change body size and shape

Disordered eating and unhealthy dieting
and distress about body size and shape

Eating disordered and disturbed body image

Larina explains that if you fall within some of these areas any activity that focuses directly on your body is going to be unpleasant. Shopping and dressing have been unpleasant and you have been precluded from developing "shopping confidence."

LACK OF SHOPPING CONFIDENCE

When you have not spent much time shopping for clothes in the past, you may not know "shopping protocol." Who do you summon to look for something in the back? How many pieces should you take into the fitting room to try on at once? How do you get a new size that you may need? These all sound like pretty basic concepts, and even if you technically know the answers, you may get uncomfortable when you are in a place that has been associated with discomfort in the past, such as a retail store.

TIP

Go with the person you know who shops best. We all know these people who have a bit of an obsession with shopping. They will love to share their love for the sport of clothes purchasing with you. Don't be afraid to ask questions. They can help even the most novice shopper and they will love it!

Don't be afraid to ask for help. Consulting with an image consultant, stylist, or personal shopper (which most stores have free of charge) can help you to look at the head-to-toe package. That is when real style begins. Buying a new suit is not really dealing with all of the issues. When women start to open up their eyes to see their entire package, the focus is off the body and on the entire look instead.

TIP

Like many things, the best way to develop confidence with shopping is to do it over and over. You do not need to spend your life savings to do this. You can get great experience by shopping without buying as well—just try things on. Plan to go into stores and try clothing on several times per week.

FEAR

Many people who have lost a good deal of weight are unsure when to go shopping for new clothes and when to discard their "fat clothes." This indecision is driven for many by fear. Larina says it is not uncommon to have a fear that you will gain weight back right after you have invested your hard-earned money in new clothes. Some people maintain a superstitious belief that if they get rid of the "plus sizes," then they will put the weight back on and no longer be able to fit into the new "little clothes," and then they will be left clothesless.

Larina notes that discarding your previous clothes means that you must buy some new clothes, which may raise a number of anxieties. Of course, shopping anxiety can crop up and your lack of shopping confidence will become apparent. As mentioned, many overweight people are comfortable blending into the shadows by wearing dark colors like black or gray. So getting rid of these "shadow suits" can be difficult, especially if you are going for new colors that will get you noticed rather than minimize your visibility.

You may fear that your weight loss is too good to be true, so you can't really believe that you can now fit into a size 8. You may fear that if you believe it, it will somehow get taken away. You may find that even though you are now a size 8, you can't believe that it is true, so you buy a size 12 or 14.

Larina has had countless Thin Club members confess their fear of putting on the too-small-size and not having it fit. It is such a horrible feeling to try to pull on a pair of pants, only to get them no farther than your knees. The fear of clothes' getting stuck is enough to keep you trying on too-big sizes after a weight loss. Larina also says that some even fear that they will rip a small- or medium-size item when they put it on, especially if they retain the overweight body image and think that they won't be able to fit into a smaller size. Some people she counsels said they were told that they need a smaller size, but that they were nervous about splitting the seam of a size 8!

WANTING IT ALL

When you're new to the shopping game, there is so much trial and error. Your first impulse is to buy anything that fits—and then you realize that you can fit into practically anything in the store! This can lead to making the wrong choices, overbuying, getting four of an item in different colors. Many overweight people—myself among them— have a tendency to "hoard," or to buy it now because it may not be there later. I used to do this with food in the past (call it Price Club syndrome), and I plead guilty,

guilty, guilty. These days, I frequently end up doing it with clothes.

"Don't grab everything in sight," urges stylist James Aguiar. "If you've been shopping all along, you might want to save yourself money and consider tailoring some of your favorite clothes to make them look like they were made for you. But not your fat clothes—they need reconstruction, not altering." James reminds Thin Club members not to spend a lot of money because, in the beginning, you're going to be experimenting a lot. He suggests fashionable, lower-priced stores like H&M, French Connection, Zara, and Club Monaco, and sales at major department stores during the "experimentation phase" to help you establish your new look.

WHO AM I NOW? DEVELOPING YOUR STYLE

By the time I took my weight off, I was beyond forty years young! As I ploughed my way through the junior departments, turning my nose up at the Ellen Tracy prim-and-proper wear in the ladies' departments and Talbots "lady clothing," it occurred to me that I was in the throes of a "missed life crisis"! Being overweight had caused me to miss my twenties. I had worn blousy figure-hiding dresses throughout my thirties, and now I wanted to find the inner me and show it to the world! No stodgy middle-age matron dresses for me! I wanted to see heads turn as I walked past a construction site! So I went through my mini-skirt stage, my outrageous runway clothing persona, and my black leather biker-chick chic look. It has taken me a while to figure out which one of those gals is the "real" me. Maybe there is a little bit of each in me, so I've got pieces in my wardrobe for each of my new personas.

TIP

List all the styles and fashions that you feel you have missed out on. Record them as they come into your mind, even if they are skimpy, like Daisy Duke shorts. Then, after each item, write a way you can get at that fashion statement without going overboard. For instance, for the Daisy Duke shorts, you can substitute mid-thigh-length shorts in the summer or a slightly above-the-knee skirt with stockings or tights in the fall.

There was a world out there beyond the black I was used to wearing because Mama said that black hides figure flaws (that "slenderizing" thing again!). Black also makes you look and feel powerful—an important thing for some people as they lose their heft and become thinner and, in some ways, more vulnerable. The stylist I had consulted before my weight loss came along with me for a post-weight-loss shopping excursion, and she pointed out styles and colors that she thought I should try. I added bronze, green, gold, and orange to my wardrobe. I didn't automatically love everything she chose for me, but having someone there to hold my hand during the initial shopping experience, not to mention a third eye to keep me from making really stupid choices, was extremely helpful.

Stylist James Aguiar suggests that when searching for the "new you" in the guise of clothing, tread cautiously. Dressing too tight can make a woman who lost weight look heavier than she actually is. (Remember the turquoise Versace jeans with loose belly skin hanging down over the vise-grip tightness around my hips?) Too sexy can be a pitfall, as it was for me that day in the lacy see-through top. The key is to be tasteful and to express yourself through your clothing choices.

"Coco Chanel used to say, after a certain age all a woman has is mystery," James reminds us. "Don't run out and expose your new body, because you may end up sending the wrong message. Be yourself. If you're a shy person, you're not going to all of a sudden put a tube top on, because that would be a disconnect with who you are. But if you're outgoing and creative, it's OK to have the fun that you probably weren't having—in a tasteful way."

TIP

Videotape yourself. You can be doing anything on the tape, but the idea is to have yourself on tape. When we watch ourselves on tape, we have a different experience because tapes are often viewed from a more objective stance. This will help you to realize your current size. Remember that the camera can add a little weight so others probably see you as thinner than you see yourself on camera.

Once the weight was significantly down, I needed to relearn how to dress. I had to figure out how to assess my post-weight-loss clothing personality. And what was the right way to approach that daunting shopping spree? First, I took a good, hard look in the mirror. When you lose weight, some things do change, but others don't—and even after a significant weight loss it took months of toning exercise and relentless cardio to shake myself into a particular size. So I suggest you look at your body. What is your overall shape? Are you long-waisted or short-waisted? Do you still have a reserve around your hips? Is your belly a little saggy with loose skin from your pre–Thin Club life? Get in touch with your overall shape.

While you are at it, determine what colors look best on you. Believe it or not, the colors you wore pre-weight-loss may not be the colors that you will gravitate to after you've lost the weight. And most important, determine your clothing "personality."

TIP

Lie down on a large piece of paper and trace your body. When finished, take a step back and look at the drawing. You might be surprised to find out that your outline looks thinner than you thought you were. Decorate the "new you" with pictures and items that say who you really are now.

PRACTICAL MATTERS

When is the right time to get rid of your old clothes and invest in a new wardrobe? I didn't wait for the scale to go down before I went on my first shopping trip. In fact, the day I started my diet, I went to Catherine's and bought myself a few nice plus-size garments. Going shopping is akin to making an investment in yourself. For me, that was not an easy thing to do, but it helped me begin my "attitude change." It was an act of reclaiming.

For years I had put everyone else first. There was no time for me, but somehow when the children needed something or my husband or mother asked me for something, I managed to find the time to go shopping for them. Making myself a priority for once was a pivotal point in my relationship with myself. In the past, I had nurtured myself with devil's food cake; now I was going to nurture myself with pretty fabrics and colors—the best I could get for the size I was then.

I decided to look good from the day I committed to joining The Thin Club, and for me this made all the difference in the world. Prior to that first shopping trip, I went to an image consultant who advised me about the right colors, styles, and jewelry that I should wear. I followed her guidelines, even took swatches with me when I went shopping. I was committing to a new lifestyle—my own extreme makeover—and I was going to look good and feel good from day one. Although I was still shopping in "fat stores," I bought myself a pair of jeans and a sweater or two that made me feel like I was en route to the "new me."

TIP

Before you start losing weight, buy a couple of good foundation undergarments. They will make you feel a bit slimmer, even though you haven't yet lost weight. They will also keep your body confined, making it difficult to comfortably overindulge—no loosening your belt buckle with a tight smoothie garment! You will be off to a great-looking and motivating start.

I also bought myself a belt—a symbolic gesture to help me rope in the fat clothes, since I knew that this time I was going to lose that weight, once and for all.

TIP

Say good-bye ceremoniously. Weight loss does technically represent a "loss." Even though most experiences are positive, there are likely to be certain aspects of your previously overweight self that you will miss. The clothing represents this previous self. Say good-bye to this chapter in your life by acknowledging the good and bad experiences you had. Once you have done so, you are ready to discard those clothes.

I got rid of most of my fat clothes as I lost the weight, but I kept one or two "hallmark" pieces that had special significance, as a reminder of just how big I once was. And those items keep looking bigger as years of living smaller go by.

James Aguiar says the time to discard your "fat clothes" is immediately. "Why hold on to things that remind you of unhappy times? To keep an entire wardrobe is too risky and easy to slip back into. If you're going to keep anything, keep just one piece to remind you of where you never want to go again." And rather than leaving the "fat clothes" around to clutter your closet, Carey Rademacher, cofounder of ItsDeductible (software that enables you to figure out how to value your IRS hidden treasures), suggests that you donate the clothing to charity. People trying to get back on their feet will value your old clothes, so not only will you be doing yourself a psychological favor, you are helping others at the same time.

TIP

Donate your plus-size clothes. Give your clothes to charity and get a tax write-off. Use the money you saved in taxes to buy yourself a couple of new essentials. If you have any very nice plus-size clothes, give them to someone you know who's trying to lose weight so that person can start dressing well while he or she loses weight.

SIZING YOURSELF UP

TIP

Try on a size too small. If you fear that it will be the most horrible experience in the world, the only way to find out is to do it. If you are now a size 10, try on a 6 or 8. Is it really the end of the world that you can't pull a 6 up? You may actually be excited to discover you are almost able to get into a size 6! Chances are that you will not rip it and will realize that it is important to try on some different sizes, even if too small.

James Aguiar says that no matter where you are in the weight-loss derby, it is essential that you try on clothes and not gauge size by eye. "When people have lost a lot of weight, they can't trust themselves to size up a rack of clothing and know what will fit," he says. "Shopping is not meant to be quick. Take the time. This may be a new experience for people who were once overweight, who breezed into a store and bought whatever happened to fit. But there are no international or even domestic sizing rules, so even a thin person just doesn't know what will fit until she or he is behind the dressing-room door."

DETERMINING WHAT YOU REALLY NEED

Because clothing costs money, and replacing an entire wardrobe is much more costly than adding an item or two each spring or fall, it is a good idea to figure out who you are and what you are most likely to need when shopping for post-weight-loss clothing. Ask yourself how much time you spend these days in exercise clothes, business clothes, "mommy" casual, rugged "weekend warrior" clothes, Sunday afternoon breezy jeans, or evening wear.

Here's a chart I used to help me go on that first significant post-weight-loss shopping spree:

CLOTHING STYLES	PERCENTAGE OF TIME SPENT
Business	_____
Evening (dinner out)	_____
Day in the park casual	_____
Rugged outdoorsy	_____
Exercise	_____
Glam social event/black tie	_____
Comfort clothes	_____
Nightclothes	_____

If you were to inspect my pre-weight-loss wardrobe and compare it to my post-weight-loss one, you'd find a number of differences. My Thin Club wardrobe features a week's worth of workout clothes. I no longer wear oversize T-shirts and baggy sweats when I go to the gym, and since every day finds me doing some form of exercise, I spend a lot of time in workout clothes. I find that wearing clean and professional workout clothes inspires me to work out harder and longer, so I keep an ample and pretty selection on hand and I wear them every day with pride! And when the clothes get ratty and worn, I discard them immediately. Exercise clothes, including binding sports bras, yoga pants with spandex that won't ride down, and good impact-absorbing sneakers are an integral part of my wardrobe.

Just as a foundation garment was the first thing I bought when I embarked on my weight loss, I continue to buy foundation garments, albeit in smaller sizes. Anyone who has carried around excess weight for any length of time is going to find that gravity tends to take over, making good foundation undergarments a necessity to help suck in the loose skin that you are likely to have unless you've invested in cosmetic surgery procedures. I make sure to keep a supply of foundation bras, girdles, and smoothies to help me look my very best and feel confident and fit.

And brrrr . . . sweaters, fleece, down, furry things, anything warm—that is what you'll find in my closet these days! Unlike my pre-weight-loss wardrobe, which found me sweating even in the most frigid conditions, my Thin Club winter wardrobe has to be really warm. My weight loss has made me very sensitive to the cold.

THE THIN CLUB SHOPPING EXPERIENCE NOW

Shopping can actually be fun once you've finally learned to accept your new body. While it's taken getting used to, these days I actually look forward to my shopping trips—and the dressing-room mirror has never looked better! I've learned to dress appropriately, blaze through stores single-mindedly searching for the right item to complete my current "look." I've learned that even though I'm thin, there are certain styles that will never look right on me, even if I lost that "last ten pounds" that I swear I will someday shed!

The most important lesson learned was to accept my new body. Once I did that, the only problem I face is finding enough money to afford the clothes that I now enjoy buying.

TWELVE

SOCIAL SITUATIONS

Handling Holidays, Parties, and Vacations

BÛCHE DE NOËL, PEPPERMINT STICKS, PUMPKIN PIE, chestnuts roasting on an open fire, stuffed mushrooms, *pâté de foie-gras,* Easter eggs with creamy centers, Valentine's Day truffles, sizzling latkes at Hanukkah and crunchy matzo on Passover—just a few of the delicacies that make the holidays, well, the holidays. And then there are the parties and the wine and the cocktails.

HOLIDAY TEMPTATIONS

So many of our festivities are centered on a bountiful table of food. And so many of our cultural events are food oriented. It is very difficult to separate ourselves from what I call the "mad rush for potato kugel" at the synagogue after-services buffet.

I laugh when I sit at my desk and see the e-mails announcing flavored popcorn, chocolate mousse cake, boxes of elegant chocolates, bagels with cream cheese, and other goodies available during the holidays, gratis, in the company cafeteria. What makes everyone rush off to the lunchroom like ladies on a shopping spree the day after

Thanksgiving? Is it because it is free—a food gift—that makes it extra-special?

I picture the cake for a minute, think about the new me, and delete the e-mail. Then again, I was never a public eater. Because I had been overweight for most of my life, I was particularly sensitive to the fact that people would be watching to see what the fat lady was eating. I also felt uncomfortable navigating my hefty body in crowded places, like around buffet tables. So when I did eat publicly, I scrupulously watched my portion sizes and made exacting food choices. This did not keep me from visiting bakeries, however, and bringing the best holiday treats home so I could gorge on them in the privacy of my own kitchen.

My holiday food battles were private ones, but some of the lessons I learned from denying myself the experience of celebrating with others in public might be helpful to those who have trouble at holiday fetes. I learned to:

• Focus on the conversation, not the menu. It was so much easier to converse, make friends, launch connections, and exchange business cards without the added concern of juggling plates, drinks, and the distractions of passing hors d'oeuvres.

• Make food a peripheral, not the center of a holiday celebration. Holidays are about spirituality, fun, friends, and family. When I am focused on food, I lose perspective in the mad rush to get the first latke. Think about the miracles you are celebrating, and the joy and the good health you have to be thankful for, and food will take a natural backstage position, where it belongs.

• Picture myself the way I'd like others to see me. It is much more elegant to spin around the party room and chat without a mouthful of pasta salad.

• Assess my choices before indulging. Many catered

meals are mirrors and lights when it comes to nutrition and taste. While the food looks amazing on a well-decorated plate, when you bite into it you realize that it just wasn't worth the calories. I learned to evaluate whether the morsel is really worth the caloric expenditure. When it is, just one taste will suffice.

• Know that I'm not missing anything by saying "No, thanks" to the holiday food. Food will always be there, and each party isn't a once-in-a-lifetime opportunity to sample a particular food. With the Internet, the Food Channel, and some great cookbooks, there is no food that I can't enjoy in moderation when I am so inclined; I don't have to have one particular item on a particular holiday, at the risk of missing it forever.

It is possible to not only handle the holidays but also enjoy them *and* not gain the weight back. Here's how.

REFOCUSING FROM FOOD TO SOCIALIZING

Contrary to popular opinion, the holidays aren't all about food. It certainly seems that way from Thanksgiving until New Year's, but if you can keep the other purposes in mind, you'll find that you're better able to keep food out of your head (and mouth).

In general, the holidays are a social time. If you find yourself far from family and friends, you can still create a social setting for yourself. You can travel to the family or friends who are easiest to get to. You can volunteer and enjoy spending time with other volunteers and the people who are grateful for what you're doing to help. You can invite people over or arrange a neighborhood caroling party. You can go to a dance and burn calories on New Year's. Basically, there are many things you can do to ensure that you are actively involved with others over the holidays.

When you're with others, you can switch the focus to socializing and away from food. The more you are actively engaged in conversation, the slower you will eat and the less you will eat. You won't think about food as much if you're keeping busy with friends and family. Be mindful of manners and not talking with your mouth full. This means that if you're involved with conversations, you can't be eating nonstop. That's a good thing! Remind yourself that you want your relationships to last, not the tempting pies and cakes to last (on your thighs). Devote yourself to your friends and family and not to the buffet table. Commit to shifting your focus of attention and choosing to limit the quantities of food that you eat.

Another great thing about the holiday season is that there are many wonderful activities that add no calories or that actually burn off calories. Get a group of friends together and walk around the neighborhood to look at holiday decorations. Go window-shopping with your brother or sister. Take your dog out to play in the snow. Go sledding or ice-skating with your kids. Spin around the dance floor.

The holidays are an excellent time to review the ideas and values that you'd like to instill in your kids. Decide whether you want all their holiday memories and traditions to be about eating, or if there are other enjoyable activities you'd like to encourage. If it's hard to do it for yourself, plan to be a role model for your children or other family members. Start some new non-food-related traditions for your family.

TIP

Make the holidays a social affair. Surround yourself with people who you enjoy; this will help reduce some of the stress of the holidays, which could lead to emotional eating. Limit your time with those who create more stress for you. When you're with others, focus on your conversations rather than the food.

WHEN FOOD ABOUNDS

One of the hardest aspects of the holidays is that food pops up when you're not ready for it. You walk into what you anticipate will be a grueling board meeting, only to find a plate of frosted gingerbread men looking up at you. You go over to a friend's house, where smells of vanilla and cinnamon are in the air. You arrive at your office starving after not having time for breakfast and are greeted by tasty, tantalizing treats.

There are three important strategies for handling these situations. The first is to be sure you are not entering them hungry. A client recently told Larina how she was running late to work and skipped breakfast one day in December. When she arrived at work, there were five boxes of donuts, two cakes, and a plate of holiday cookies in the office kitchen. More than ever, the holidays are a time to eat regular, healthy, well-balanced meals and not to walk around hungry. It is just too easy to grab something filled with sugar and starch and to get caught up in a series of sugar highs and lows. Instead, be sure you are having plenty of proteins, fiber, fruits, and vegetables.

The second strategy for handling these situations is to remove yourself from them. If you walk into your office kitchen and you see an array of fattening foods, turn around and leave. In psychology, this is called *stimulus control,* which means that you control your environment to help you break an unhelpful habit. Keep out of the fattening zones—you know, the areas where you can gain five pounds just from standing there. If this is impossible, keep yourself in another part of the room.

Likewise, be sure that you don't have cookies, cakes, and other goodies in your home or office. If you decide to enjoy a holiday treat, take just one and then remove yourself from the situation so it is difficult to take more. Or, keep your hands full with a glass of water and hold your purse or something else, so they aren't able to pick up snacks. Grazing is a major source of holiday weight gain or regain, so be aware of what you select to eat.

A third strategy is to look for ways to create delicious holiday food that is also healthy and low in fat. It can be a fun challenge to look for new ways to avoid fats when you bake. Great cookbooks out there can help you with this process. You can, for example, create high-fiber (with wheat germ added), low-fat (substitute applesauce for oil) blueberry muffins that are a scrumptious breakfast or snack. Always look for healthy alternatives for you and your family. Gingerbread cookies, for example, are often better than sugar cookies. When you use this strategy in combination with portion control (eat one small gingerbread man, not the entire gingerbread extended family), you will avoid feeling deprived and will reinforce the idea that you can make treats more healthful with a little effort. So,

- Don't walk around hungry!
- Remove yourself from temptation.
- Keep your holiday cuisine healthy and portion controlled.

TIP

Play the "lighten it up" game and see how good you can be at creating healthy alternatives. Organize a group of friends who are interested in losing or maintaining weight and who are invested in healthy eating. Get together twice a month to exchange your healthy recipes at a potluck supper.

Most important, don't let your fear of fat ruin your enjoyment of holidays. Many formerly overweight people experience a peak in anxiety during holidays because they fear the food. Don't let fear take away your fun! Remind yourself what the holidays are really about, use the strategies outlined above, practice moderation and portion control, and realize that you can enjoy the holidays and not gain weight.

PARTY POLITICS

Parties can be intimidating for a former fat person. Food and drink aside, being decked out in your "party best" and thrust into a room of vibrating, hip-grinding people can be scary. Did I dress appropriately? How do I compare to other people in the room? Am I older or younger than they are? Am I prettier or more handsome? Do I look stupid on the dance floor? For a shy person who was used to hiding behind a "fat persona," negotiating the holiday party took some relearning. Is it any wonder that most people can't handle a party without some degree of inebriation?

Anyone raised in New York City, or any other urban area, for that matter, has been conditioned to never meet the eyes of a stranger. Discretion is essential for safety reasons. At a party, however, you are required to undo the conditioning, cruise the room, and catch someone's eye and smile to get the person's attention! Not easy. If you were a former "life of the party" fat person who joked about your weight, food, and appearance, you also might have some adjustment problems. People are looking at you differently now. You've gone from "There's Fred, the Fat Guy—let's see if he's got a couple of good jokes for us" to "Hey, is that Fred? Looking hot!" from the women. And colleagues may see you as someone they don't necessarily want to be standing too close to, lest you steal their limelight or their coveted promotion. The holiday party can become a turf war.

OWNING THE ROOM

So how does Fred the Fat Guy morph into Fred the Party Animal? And how does Formerly Fatricia turn into the woman everyone wants to talk to? First, say yes to parties. Even if your initial inclination is to run the other way, say you'll go.

Before the party, eliminate the negative chatter in your head. Change "I hate parties!" into "I am going to have a great time!" Instead of worrying about being a wallflower, decide that you will say hello to just one new person (male or female). Allow yourself one drink (no more) to loosen up, if that's what you need. Prepare just one conversational item that's simple to repeat to everyone you meet. The holiday theme can work for you—your impending holiday plans or upcoming vacation can be great conversation topics.

TIP

Get into the party mindset. Remind yourself how parties are fun, how you can meet new people, and how great you'll feel afterward. Don't dwell on all the things that could go wrong. Instead, focus on all the things that could go well.

As for the pulsating room, if you are ill at ease and frightened at first, know that you're not alone. Many people find parties intimidating. But see it as an opportunity, not a burden. Start with a "third-person" approach. Pretend you are a news reporter surveying the party. Map out the territory. Food tables are due east. Bar due west. Coat check in the corner. Observe the way other people are looking at each other, cruising the room, flirting, bumping, grinding, or drunk and letting their inhibitions run wild. Look for some of the successful schmoozers and watch their body language.

When you have the lay of the land, put on your best attitude. You are fabulous! Walk with confidence across the party floor, knowing that you are a great-looking, interesting person and you have made a remarkable transformation. Anyone in this room would be better off for having talked to you, danced with you, smiled at you! You're not fat anymore—no need to hide behind a jocular façade or a table loaded with goodies. You are sexy, smart, fit, and fun. Mingle, meet, greet, and enjoy.

NAVIGATING VACATIONS

The same frenzy to "taste it all" used to follow me around on vacation, making the vacation more about the next meal than about enjoying the sights, sounds, and activities that the places offered. Some vacations, like hotels in the Catskills, were all about the next meal. Even though they had tennis, golf, ice-skating, and bicycle riding, my husband and I would fret that we would be late for a meal. That fear would totally wreck our activity schedule. Were we afraid we would starve if we missed that meal? I guess so. And what a meal it was; with as many carb- and fat-laden entrees as desired from the menu and little "noshes" that the waitress would slip to you in the hopes of receiving a hefty tip. It was a bloat-fest!

Naturally, as I lost weight, my idea of a dream vacation changed radically. My last vacation took me to Israel. I brought my protein shakes for breakfast and passed by the outrageous breakfast buffets that were an add-on at the hotel. I didn't need pastries, breads, and carbs for breakfast. If I wanted to sample the local fare, I treated myself to a falafel (sans the pita) at lunch, with plenty of deliciously fresh organic Israeli salad. The local produce was intoxicating and low in calories.

Instead of wasting all that time loading up my plate, I challenged myself to run up the snake path at Masada. I rappelled down a breathtaking crater at Mitzpeh Ramon, climbed chalk cliffs at Sdei Boker, and kayaked on tributaries of the Jordan River in the Golan Heights. And when I wasn't looking for fun activities with kids in tow, I was downstairs at the hotel gym running on the treadmill with weights in hand or running with my wrist weights up and down the Jerusalem Hills. Did I work up an appetite? You bet I did! And did I indulge? In healthy delicious food, absolutely! I veered away from the fatty, sugary stuff. "Just one rugelach," my son begged me. "It's the marzipan kind—you'll never taste it again." Says who? If I don't catch it this time around, it will be here waiting for me next time. And even though I said no to the rugelach, it was the best vacation I ever had. I saw more than I used to, worried less about meal planning, and focused on the things that matter on vacation, such as seeing the sites and having once-in-a-lifetime experiences unique to a particular location.

Are you one of the many people who worry about traveling and gaining weight? It is often difficult to maintain your lifestyle of healthy eating when you're on vacation; you need to eat out, and there may not be healthy snacking options nearby. It's also tough because you have the "on vacation" mentality, and it's easy to make excuses to treat yourself. Because of these challenges, some people avoid going on vacations. Others gain some of their weight back. And some find vacations to be stressful because of those food-choice worries. Don't be one of these people. Enjoy your much-earned vacation without worrying about food or gaining weight back; just increase your activities and make good food choices.

Heavy people are often limited in what they can do on vacation. Now that you are thin, you might find yourself with more activities to try than you ever fathomed—for instance, scuba diving, cliff climbing, or just going on certain rides at Six Flags that were prohibited when you were heavy. Rejoice in this new freedom and push yourself to try some new things, even those that are nerve-wracking. So, make a list of all the vacations and activities that you didn't do when you were heavy. If some of them look intimidating, begin with ones that seem more reasonable and work your way up to the wild ones. Find an adventurous friend or family member to travel with.

One of the benefits to creating a vacation around recreation is that you will be active while you travel. Your trip won't be centered on eating and drinking. You'll be so busy doing everything that you won't have much time to eat. And you'll have burned off so many calories with a half-day hike, a long run on the beach, or an adventurous kayaking trip that you can enjoy some great food, as well. Even if you're not on a trip with much opportunity for activity, you can always hit the hotel pool or fitness center.

TIP

Plan calorie-burning activities during your vacation. Give yourself enjoyable things to look forward to instead of the all-you-can-eat dinners, and get exercise in while you travel.

In addition to increasing your activities while on vacation, be mindful of your food choices. Plan ahead for your trip. Pack some healthy snacks such as dried fruits, nuts, wheat crackers, and granola bars. Bring some whole-grain cereal for breakfast and get milk when you arrive at your destination. You'll also save money by bringing your own snacks and breakfasts.

For dinner, reduce the portion size by sharing meals or ordering a half portion, even if you have to pay full price. Many people object to this idea because they feel that it is wasting money. But ask yourself: What do you value more, the money or your weight loss? Remember that you'll be spending the same amount of money, so you aren't really wasting money. Plus, you'll waste less food because the kitchen will prepare less for you. Once you've received the nourishment and hunger-reducing value from the food, you don't need to eat any more. You won't get any more benefit from eating a gigantic plate of pasta than you would by eating one-half or one-third of it. In the long run, "wasting" the food or money will save you money and keep you healthy.

TIP

Watch portions especially carefully during holidays and vacations. Because you will have all kinds of fattening and tempting foods around you, you need to be prepared. Don't skip meals, fill up on foods with fiber, drink extra water, and watch the portion sizes. If you're at a restaurant and have finished half your meal, ask the server to take the plate away and drink water as your dining mates finish their meals. And be sure to avoid all-you-can-eat and all-inclusive situations.

"YOU LOOK GREAT!"

How to Accept Compliments

"DON'T YOU LOOK AMAZING! YOU HAVE LOST SO much weight! What a great dress!" And my reply?

"Yes, but it's a little tight. I still have another ten pounds to go." Why is it so hard to just say thanks to compliments? Maybe it sounds easy, but when you have been living life as a fat person, you're likely to find ways to deflect the admiration.

BASKING IN THE GLOW

Why is it important to bask in compliments? You've probably heard that it's a good idea to accept compliments rather than refute them, but you may not be sure exactly why. We've talked about how what you focus on often becomes your reality. If you focus on flaws and point them out to others, you will create a negative experience for yourself, draw more attention to your perceived "flaws," and possibly make these problems worse. When you focus on flaws, you sap your confidence and motivation, making it more likely that you'll regain the weight or not lose the last ten pounds.

If, on the other hand, you allow yourself to focus on your accomplishments and bask in the glow of all your hard work, you'll draw your attention to success rather than to failures. You'll feel better and continue on your path to success with weight management. Your self-esteem will improve, and you'll allow yourself to see your worthwhile and important qualities that previously were masked.

Another result is that people will treat you differently and see you differently. Compare these two responses to a compliment that someone looks great in a new T-shirt:

1. "Well, my arms are jiggling out the top here and it's a bit tight around the stomach area."
2. "Thanks, it was fun to shop and get some new clothes and I feel great!"

Notice the difference? Who would be more enjoyable to be around? If you take a closer look at the first person versus the second, what do you notice? Who do you view as more attractive? With the first person, you notice all the problems she pointed out. That is, you might not notice them at first, but when she points them out, you can't help but notice. With the second person, you notice her exuberance and glow. When you bask in the glow, others see it as well.

Even more important, the person who said the first response is likely to get fewer compliments in the future. Since she advertises her "flaws," people will notice them. Because she doesn't present herself confidently, people will not treat her as a confident and secure person. Insecure people tend to attract other insecure people, so she'll find herself surrounded by self-doubting or unstable individuals. People are more likely to take advantage of her or treat her with disrespect because she doesn't show respect for herself. In turn, she will lose confidence and have poorer self-esteem. Wow, who knew it was *so* important to accept compliments? It is!

The second woman will attract people who appreciate her and enjoy her enthusiasm. People will typically see her as confident and will treat her with respect. In turn, she will pay more attention to her positive qualities and will gain self-esteem. Beware that some people (particularly insecure or controlling people) may feel threatened by her confidence and attempt to shoot her down. These are the type of people who sabotage your Thin Club membership, and you may choose to disassociate with them.

TIP

Get more compliments by handling compliments graciously. When you get more compliments, you start to feel better about yourself, and when you feel better about yourself, you get more compliments. Help yourself and others to see your strengths and positive qualities rather than your flaws.

WHY IT'S HARD TO ACCEPT COMPLIMENTS

Why are former fat people likely to shy away from compliments? There are many reasons. First, you may not believe the compliment. As we've discussed throughout the book, your self-concept doesn't just change overnight when the weight comes off. While you may know that you look different, you may not feel different. You, or at least part of you, may still believe that you look fat. You may be skeptical about any compliments and think that people are saying them just to be nice.

Second, you may be used to rejecting compliments. Whether you believe it or not, you have a learned response of shying away from compliments or pointing out why they aren't true. Habits are hard to break.

Third, you may be superstitious or suspicious. You might feel that it's bad luck to accept compliments, as if your accepting them makes them unlikely to stay true. Many people believe that it's not a good idea to agree with something if it isn't 100 percent true, or that they could sabotage themselves by agreeing with compliments. Others are suspicious of people who give compliments. Before you lost weight, you may have felt invisible or, worse, felt judged or under scrutiny. Now, you receive attention and compliments that you aren't used to. You wonder what that person's ulterior motive is. You think that the individual can't be genuine or you feel annoyed that nobody complimented you when you were heavier.

TIP

Assume the best in people unless you have reason to believe otherwise. Take the "innocent until proven guilty" stance, and assume that people really mean what they say when they give you a compliment.

LEARNING TO SAY THANKS

In order to be comfortable accepting compliments, you need to get them. The key is that you attract compliments and then respond in such a way that you'll get more of them. So, to get compliments in the first place, give them to yourself. When you draw your attention to your positive characteristics and attributes, you will feel great. When you feel great, you'll radiate that and others will pick up on it. One of Larina's clients tried this technique after losing fifteen pounds—less than half of her goal weight loss. Because she radiated confidence, others began complimenting her. People she'd never met before gave her compliments. And it wasn't just about the weight loss, it was about the confidence and energy she projected.

TIP

Write down three compliments to yourself every day. Putting compliments in writing is more difficult and also more compelling. This technique will also help you on those "blah" days when you're feeling particularly unattractive or unmotivated.

Once you begin receiving compliments from others, the most important thing you can do is to accept them. When you shoot someone down for giving you a compliment, how likely is it you'll get another one? You'll create a self-fulfilling prophecy and say to yourself, "See, the compliment wasn't really true. They never said it again!" But in reality, they didn't give you another compliment because of how you responded to the first one.

The most important part of gracefully accepting compliments is to resist the urge to say it isn't true. For a while, you will think that the favorable statement is completely off base—this is OK. Do *not,* however, verbalize this thought. Over time, as you *don't* say something to reflect your self-critical thoughts, they will lessen. You can change your thoughts by your behaviors, so choose to not act on those critical thoughts.

Simply smile and say, "Thank you." It is as easy as that.

If you slip up and say something unflattering, don't worry—you can make up for it. If someone who you know well gave you that compliment, tell the friend, "I need to work on accepting compliments. Thanks for what you said about me; it does make me feel good," or "I guess we're our own harshest critics, but I really appreciate your comment."

TIP

Always accept compliments, and if you accidentally shoot one down, make up for it. If it's too tough for you to accept the compliment fully at first, respond by saying, "Thanks for your interest" or "Thanks for your kind words." These responses feel a little less like you're agreeing with the flattering remark (which many say is the hardest part) yet they still acknowledge the other person for having given you the praise.

Another useful exercise is to give a lot of compliments yourself. Observe how others respond to them. How do you feel and react when someone dismisses your compliment? What do you think when the person points out the reasons it's not true? And what happens when someone graciously accepts your compliment? What do you think about that person? Are you likely to compliment the person and notice those positive attributes again?

When you try this experiment and give compliments to others, you'll see how the other shoe fits. You'll develop empathy for others and not want to make them feel bad. This may inspire you to try to say thank you, even if it's difficult to do so!

TIP

Give out compliments, tributes, and random acts of kindness. Be sincere. If you like someone's shirt, say so. If you found a friend's smile heartwarming, let her know. Learn how others respond and then try out these responses on others to see which feel most comfortable.

FOURTEEN

THE SKINNY ON SEX

WHAT IS SEXIER—FAT OR THIN? DOES SEX GET BET-ter as the pounds melt away? These questions intrigued most of my friends, who took me aside and asked me qui-etly, "How does your husband like the new you?" And of course, after I left my husband, there was all kinds of spec-ulation as to just how good sex had gotten. Was there another man?

I didn't leave for another man. And I didn't leave be-cause I got thin and sexy. The truth is, when I was sup-posedly happily married and fat, I heard more complaints outside the bedroom from my husband about my fat than I did inside the bedroom. For example, he told me that he was embarrassed being seen in public with me. He didn't like going on vacation with me when I was wearing a bathing suit. I had no energy and no inclination to exercise with him. I was a stick in the mud and I hated my own body, which didn't make me any more attractive to him, naturally.

Yet, after I lost weight, while he very much enjoyed the way others looked at me, while he wore me on his arm like a Rolex, he seemed to resent the time, attention, and money I lavished on myself. Manicures, waxing, new clothing, sexy underwear—the more focused I became on giving to myself, the more unhappy he became about the new me. And after a while, I started noticing admiring glances from other men, which delighted me and infuriated him.

Naturally, as I lost the weight, our sexual relationship went through a metamorphosis along with our marital relationship. Did my weight loss ruin my marriage? The short answer is no—it did not. Did my seizing control of my life give me the strength and control to reevaluate my marriage and leave? Absolutely! Was the tenacious balance of our sex life affected? Without a doubt!

As a newly evolving thin divorcee, I am finding that on some level I am learning to live and love again. Losing the weight made me realize that a lifetime had gone by and I never had a really healthy relationship. Although I have yet to find the ultimate experience, I can only imagine that sex must be wonderful when you have a complete physical, emotional, and spiritual connection. That means giving and taking, trusting and surrendering. That means conquering not just the layers of fat but also the painful emotional barriers that separate couples from one another. Bringing those barriers down has got to be the most powerful sexual and emotional connection anyone can ever experience. And if there's one thing I aspire to do as a new member of The Thin Club, it is to find the right person and finally experience that connection, once and for all. Because I deserve it—every bit of it, the whole nine yards!

Sexual "success" is not just about having a lean, sexy body. The body may have all the right working parts, but if the mind is not in synch with your new body, there will be no sparks in the bedroom. Anyone who has lost a significant amount of weight will confront unique intimacy and body and relationship issues; in this chapter, we'll address them.

REDISCOVERING YOUR SEXUALITY

My friend Janet had been about 125 pounds overweight for fifteen years. Her husband left her ten years before, claiming that she was not the woman he had married. Indeed, her wedding picture featured a svelte and gorgeous bride with a beaming groom. When her two children turned sixteen and eighteen, respectively, something snapped and Janet started herself on a radical diet and exercise regime. "I realized that I had been eating cookies, candy, and rice because, on some level, I missed having sex. It had been years since I had been with a man. As soon as I dropped the first forty pounds, I knew I was craving something better than sugar. And I was determined to enjoy it again."

The big question for Janet was how. She had taken herself off the market as a sexual being for so many years, and even though she was everyone's favorite confidant and had earned a reputation as one of the more sociable soccer moms, she realized that she was out of practice when it came to attracting men. Her teenagers had come to see her as anything but sexual, since for years she had lounged around in comfort clothes—ripped nighties, worn sweatshirts, and ratty elastic-waist pants. Imagine their shock when the "new" Janet slipped herself into size 12 jeans and a tight-fitting tank top. Janet enrolled herself in an online dating service, and when her children went away to be counselors at an overnight summer camp, she gingerly began dating again. "At first it was difficult," she confided. "It had been years since I'd been touched or kissed. I was nervous as a kid who was anticipating her first kiss, and I realized that my kids probably had more kissing experience in the past couple of years than I'd had in the past ten!" She met and dated several men before she found one who became her steady boyfriend. "Once I got past the scary stuff, the insecurities about not being at my goal weight and some of the flabby skin, the sex turned out to be better than great—he loved my body and I love it, too. I've rediscovered sex and it's never been better!"

THE FOOD-SEX TRADE-OFF

Food is frequently a substitute for sex—almost inter-changeable. You don't have to hunt food down or hope to get its attention at a singles bar. It doesn't jilt us or reject or argue with us. It is always there when we need it. It is a faithful partner that makes us feel good. And when we overindulge, we feel bad. That same chocolate ice cream that we use to assuage our dignity when we're craving something more sensual can obstruct our ability to un-leash our libido.

When a husband and wife are having trouble in the bedroom, one might gain weight, perhaps out of emotional angst or even with a subconscious motive. Eating, accord-ing to Barbara Bartlik, a psychiatrist who specializes in sexu-ality issues, is a solitary, oftentimes passive-aggressive activity that can be a way of saying, "You cannot control me! This is one thing that only I can control." So even if an overweight person *feels* out of control while eating, the sit-uation may be a desperate effort to control a relationship that has holes—in and out of the bedroom.

According to Cynthia Sass, a dietitian and the coauthor of *Your Diet Is Driving Me Crazy: When Food Conflicts Get in the Way of Your Love Life,* when you overeat or eat a heavy, high-fat meal, a large percentage of your blood flow goes to your digestive system, making it difficult to engage in any kind of physical activity. Add a few extra bagels and you're ready for sleepyland, not hot tantric sex. That's because high-carbohydrate meals increase serotonin levels, creating a calm, relaxing, sleepy feeling. And anything you have digested that your body cannot burn or use will be stored as fat. A huge meal is stored as fat, putting additional stress on all of your organs, joints, and muscles, creating more wear and tear, even during the most pleasurable physical activity. When you overeat, it's uncomfortable. At that point, says Cynthia, people learn to "disconnect" from their body, making it virtually impossible to experience the gamut of pleasurable, body-focused, sexual feelings and taking away the energy or drive for sex.

In addition, most people do not feel at their most attractive when they have a full belly. Put together the physical and emotional components, and overeating is not a recipe for a strong libido. When your togetherness as a couple centers on food (going out to eat or eating large meals at home), you may be sabotaging the sexual and romantic aspects of your relationship.

HORMONAL CHANGES

Do you need to be athletic and lithe and able to execute sexual acrobatics to enjoy the ultimate orgasm? Certainly not. But according to Christine Ren, a surgeon at NYU Medical Center, when someone loses a massive amount of weight, it changes the landscape of the estrogen, progesterone, and testosterone levels in the body. In women, fat cells retain estrogen, that nice hormone that partners with testosterone to lube you up and make you feel sexy. Weight changes can alter menstrual patterns in women and sexual libido in both men and women, especially immediately after a weight loss. After the fat cells shrink and a person has been thin for a while, the hormone levels tend to normalize.

IMPROVED SELF-IMAGE

Fat is insulation. Fat is a barrier. A big belly and cellulite thighs provide a buffer between two people when they hug and cling to one another. Does sex feel better when you're thin or when you are fat? Sex feels better when your self-image is intact. It is wonderful to know that you can let go, be without inhibitions about belly fat and love handles, and—oh, my God—what is he thinking when he really looks at me without my clothes? But as we discussed throughout this book, being thin now does not necessarily mean you are automatically in synch with your sexy body. Self-image is something that needs to be perfected in order for you to have uninhibited, tantric, miraculous, spirited, and spiritual sex.

"The greater cause of increased libido after a large weight loss is the increased self-esteem," Dr. Ren explains. "That combines with the fact that someone who is thin is more likely to get more sexual attention than his or her heavy counterpart. The added bonus is less shortness of breath during sexual activity. And without that belly-fat cushion in between the two partners, sex becomes more pragmatic, and ultimately more enjoyable."

TIP

Loser wins lingerie! Have your partner buy you (or if you are single, buy yourself) a new piece of lingerie to celebrate each ten pounds and/or each new definition line you see in your muscular new body! It's a sexy way of celebrating your continued success on the scale *and* in the bedroom!

GETTING IN THE MOOD

According to Dr. Bartlik, it is no secret that estrogen is stored in fat cells. That is why perimenopausal women who are overweight tend to be spared hot flashes. Testosterone, which is necessary for drive, arousal, and orgasm, tends to follow the estrogen cycle, which explains why there are certain "spikes" in women's desire at specific times during her menstrual cycle. There is no doubt that shrinking fat cells deplete a body's estrogen supply. But according to Dr. Bartlik, sexuality is 50 percent brain and 50 percent body. Simply stated, if you are not in a good mindset about your sexuality, you can turn it around by putting yourself in the mood.

The cycle, according to Dr. Bartlik, goes something like this:

Low self-esteem → Eat → Gain weight →
Feel bad about body → Can't "let go" during
sex → Lack of enjoyment during sex → Partner
cools off because he/she isn't enjoying sex →
Heavy person experiences loss because of
partner's disinterest → Heavy person experiences
low self-esteem → Cycle begins again.

To break the cycle, Dr. Bartlik suggests that you focus on the part of yourself that is sexy: accentuate the good. In fact, if you can, she suggests that rather than thinking about your body as you approach a sexual encounter, you engage in a fantasy. As you get more aroused, your sexual partner will have heightened arousal. And the above cycle will be reversed.

She recommends that patients set the tone for sex by creating a sensual scenario that takes the focus off your physical self and shifts it to the environment. Appealing to each of the five senses sets the sexual "stage." Begin with aroma, she suggests. Light scented candles to waft in lavender or vanilla—fragrances that evoke sensuality, according to studies. Wear sensual fabrics like silk, cashmere, or fur to bring "tingle" to bed with you. Set the lights carefully and make your environment visually appealing. As hackneyed as some romantic music might be, she suggests putting on something that brings you to "that place." And then there is the sense of taste. For that she recommends chocolate—in moderation, of course—since it has been shown to have aphrodisiac effects. Rosie, my weight-loss guru, says an occasional square of dark chocolate, 60 percent or more, is perfectly OK and can quell chocolate cravings, so by all means, don't be afraid to indulge. If all goes well, you will be working it off in the most sexual exercise of all.

TIP

Indulge the five senses. Use your senses to get you out of your internal critic and self-consciousness and into the mood. Develop mindfulness skills to fully experience the situation at hand, being completely present in the moment and not in your head in an internal dialogue. Notice the sites, smells, temperature, textures, tastes, and sounds as you experience them prior to intimacy, which will help get you in the mood and help keep you in the mood.

EVALUATING YOUR RELATIONSHIPS

"I can't divorce him. I'm too fat—who will look at me?" one friend, miserable in her marriage, confided. When you were heavy, you may have had such insecurities about your body that kept you in an unsatisfactory or even an abusive relationship. So what happens now that you've lost the weight? You might have expected a sudden increase in confidence and willingness to leave a dead-end relationship. For some this happens, and for others it doesn't.

Losing weight may give you the boost in self-assurance you need to realize that you are worth more than a lousy relationship. The boost in energy and serotonin that results from regular exercise has improved your mood. Your well-balanced eating and reduced consumption of unhealthy sugars and caffeine has decreased your anxiety and put you in a more balanced mood. Compliments have given the old ego a little stroke, especially when you take them well, as we discussed in the last chapter. New friends, activities, and support systems remind you that there's no reason to stay in an unfulfilling relationship. As a result, you look at your relationship from a new perspective. This new outlook can make you evaluate your relationship more positively *or* more negatively.

STAY? OR MOVE ON?

If you realize that your relationship is improved when you feel and look better, you'll likely decide to stay in it. You might find that you feel more secure with yourself and that makes you more secure in the relationship. Your sexual relationship can improve also as you become more focused on your significant other and less focused on whether your thighs are jiggling or your stomach is appropriately hidden. You may feel closer to your partner if he or she has been supportive during your weight-loss challenge. Your partner's love and encouragement has helped you stay on track and lose the weight. Or maybe you lost the weight together.

While these positive results can certainly occur, it is equally possible that you will see your relationship in a more negative light and will think about ending it. You might realize that the relationship has been less than satisfactory all along or that some negative changes occurred after weight loss that you are not happy about. Some people say that their partners suddenly become possessive, jealous, or controlling after they've lost weight. They have not been used to your receiving attention from others and they feel threatened by it. If this is the case, realize that your partner's reactions are normal, but there are certain behaviors that are unacceptable and can lead to a miserable or abusive relationship. If your significant other shows a bit of jealousy, try to be understanding and supportive, and let him or her know that there is no need for worry. If, on the other hand, your partner begins putting you down, keeping constant tabs on you, or restricting your activities, realize that these controlling behaviors are often the first steps to an abusive relationship. If you spot verbally abusive or controlling behaviors, you may want to consult with the National Domestic Violence Hotline, 1-800-799-SAFE (7233).

If you decide to move on, you may feel empowered by your new body and lifestyle. You know that you can accomplish what you set out to do because you've accomplished another major success that was challenging (your weight loss). You have overcome a huge obstacle, so you can risk being out on your own and entering the intimidating dating world.

You may have ambivalence about staying in the relationship. One client, Jen, told Larina, "My husband loved me even when I was fat and was supportive of my weight loss. He's a good man and I feel bad about lacking a physical attraction to him. How horrible it would be to leave him as soon as I'm thin and more desirable to other men!" Her guilt kept her in a relationship that she'd been ready to leave for a while.

Jen had hoped that her sexual relationship with her husband would improve once she'd lost the weight. She thought maybe it was her own insecurities and discomfort with her body. But it wasn't, and her sexual chemistry with her husband didn't improve. After she lost the weight, she was more comfortable with her body but not with her husband. In reality, they never had a sexual chemistry. Her initial decision to marry him was partly influenced by a fear that she would never achieve intimacy with someone, and she seized the opportunity to be with a nice man who treated her well. You can imagine how Jen struggled with her desire to leave her husband. He supported her for many years and she felt ungrateful and guilty about her decision that they would never have the intimacy she longed for.

If you do not know for sure that you are ready to move on, then give yourself a little post-weight-loss time to think about it. In making major life decisions, it is often wise to postpone decisions (when possible) during times of significant transition. Your mind is not in a stable place, and you may make snap or rushed decisions that you could later regret.

As you can see, there are many potential changes that can occur within your love relationships following a weight loss. Do not judge yourself for having any particular reaction, and try not to be too surprised if your reaction wasn't what you expected. Like many new things, it's hard to predict how you'll feel until you're in the situation. Give it a little time, think about what you really want or value in a relationship, talk with supportive people in your life, and the right decision will come to you.

TIP

Consider your relationship pre-post. List the positive qualities about your relationship before and after the weight loss and do the same for the negative qualities. Ideally, you will want to see some positive characteristics that have been consistent throughout your relationship to show that your partner loves you for yourself. If you can't come up with several key positive characteristics about your relationship before and after weight loss, you could have a problem. Of course it is possible, even likely, that your significant other will become more attracted to you after your weight loss, but you'll want to feel that he or she loves you for more than your thin new body.

If you list many new, negative qualities, talk to your significant other about these changes. Realize that there may be an adjustment period, but determine where you will draw the line, and choose to end the relationship if things don't improve.

FIFTEEN

LOOSE ENDS

Plastic Surgery

I WAS GETTING READY FOR A PHOTO SHOOT. A woman's magazine had looked at my "befores" and "afters" and was so impressed that they wanted to feature me as a weight-loss success story. They chose my clothing, carefully blew out my hair, and applied my makeup. A stylist walked in surveying me critically as I stood in my red cashmere sweater and tight-fitting yoga pants.

I was sleek. I was thin. She shook her head sadly and stared at my chest. "The breasts are the first things to go when you lose weight, eh?"

Hmph! I had been a 42D in my "former life." I was down to a 34C. I wasn't filling out that sweater enough to look sexy for the photo shoot. At that moment I didn't know which was more deflated—my breasts or my ego. I had worked hard to get where I was, and I was finally acknowledging my thin self, but it appeared that I'd reached the end of what I could control.

I no longer hate the sight of me naked in front of the mirror. I've worked hard to tone myself and it certainly shows. And, yes, I look better naked at my age than I did in my twenties and thirties. But deflated breasts, a belly riddled with stretch marks, loose skin enveloping that last little pouch of fat cells that droops when I do my push-ups, and big arms are the remnants of years and years of being a fat girl, of aging (albeit slowly), and God's gift to me from my grandma. I do envy women with smooth and supple bellies, sleek and lean arms, and full, perky breasts. I know that for every woman with a perfect body, there are ten more who are battling the ravages of bulges and sags. Skin elasticity, genetics, and age are major factors in the ultimate appearance of a body. However, we have a few choices:

• We can do as our mothers did, and buy a very strong girdle and long-line bra with whalebones to put everything where it should be. The downside of this is that nowadays we tend to bare a lot more (even as we get "older") than we did when Jacqueline Kennedy was First Lady. All the girdles in the world won't help you during bikini and tank-top season!

• We can continue to do our Pilates and toning exercises, praying that eventually everything will somehow spring into shape, or at least we'll look better in spandex and bared at the beach.

• We can acknowledge our wonderful accomplishments, ignore the bulges and hanging skin, and dress carefully in the summer to accentuate the positive and de-emphasize the negative; and at some point say, "To hell with it all—I earned my sags and I'm going to wear them with pride!"

• We can visit plastic surgeons and ask them if they can help us complete the job we started.

- We can visit bariatric physicians and get recommendations for spot fat reduction.

Whatever our choices, we should be careful not to judge one another. As Thin Club members we have already chosen to improve our lives significantly, and every member deserves a big pat on the back for joining and staying in The Thin Club. Whether you are in the "love yourself no matter what" group or the "fine-tune the body with help from modern medicine" group, there should be acceptance and acknowledgment of the awesome job we have all done to look and feel our best, and to extend our lives by being healthy.

WHERE YOU'RE MOST LIKELY TO NEED A NIP (OR TUCK)

Andrew Kleinman, a board-certified plastic surgeon by the American Board of Plastic Surgeons, in private practice in Westchester County, New York, has built a career around making people feel better about their bodies, using reconstruction and cosmetic surgery. He says a person who has lost a lot of weight is often surprised by the residual hanging folds of skin. "It can take the joy out of what is by all means a major accomplishment," says Dr. Kleinman.

According to Dr. Kleinman, the best time for cosmetic surgery is after you have lost weight and your new weight has been stable for three to six months. If you are not yet stable in your weight loss and have surgery, you may find that after losing more than another ten pounds, you will end up with loose skin again. Touch-ups are costly. Also, if you gain weight after your surgery, you may stretch your skin and cause skin damage or stretch marks. So how do you know if you need to lose more weight or if what you are left with is hanging skin? Dr. Kleinman says the rule of thumb is, "If it hangs, it's skin." When you are left with hanging skin, building up your muscles will never shrink the skin. So, chances are, if you've lost a lot of weight and are staring at pouches that don't seem to tighten even when you "suck in," it's loose skin.

Areas of the body most likely to be affected by weight loss include:

ABDOMEN

The lower abdomen is the most common area to be affected by weight loss. It is the lowest point, Dr. Kleinman says, where everything hangs.

The Cosmetic Fix

In patients who have had bariatric procedures, when there is documentation of health problems that include rashes, skin problems, yeast and bacterial infections, or interference in going to the bathroom (which happens more frequently with men), insurance companies sometimes pay for *panniculectomy,* a limited procedure that amputates the excess skin of the lower abdomen. The other procedure, usually not covered by insurance, is *abdominoplasty* (i.e., tummy tuck), a procedure that generally includes redistributing the skin of the entire abdomen, sometimes including tightening the muscles by putting sutures in the fascia on top of the muscle. Both panniculectomy and abdominoplasty can be combined with *liposuction* to achieve even results. The most extreme abdominal contouring surgery is called *belt lipectomy,* also not covered by most insurance companies. It involves removing the skin of the lower abdomen and attaching the upper torso to the lower torso at the bikini line.

Panniculectomy and abdominoplasty can be done on

an outpatient basis, with the patient often going home the same day. The surgery takes between one and four hours and patients are generally able to go back to nonstrenuous activities within a week. The scars are tucked away in the bikini line. A belt lipectomy, on the other hand, is a six- to twelve-hour procedure that may require blood transfusions. The recovery requires up to three days in the hospital, and the patient is generally not able to resume regular activities for weeks afterward.

BREASTS

Women who have lost a lot of weight tend to end up with an empty skin envelope where their breasts once were. That, combined with the drooping that gravity brings to women as they age, can be pretty demoralizing to someone expecting a bathing-beauty body post-weight-loss. Men who have lost significant amounts of weight can end up with loose skin on their breasts as well. As in a drooping abdomen, men and women with hanging skin in the breast area can end up with skin ailments.

The Cosmetic Fix

Mastopexy, also known as breast lift, is a surgery frequently used to eliminate the loose skin. The male breast reduction is called *gynecomastia,* and it reduces enlarged breasts using liposuction and/or cutting out excess glandular tissue. In some states, this is covered by insurances, in post-bariatric procedures, depending on how many grams are removed from the breast. According to Dr. Kleinman, the surgery can be augmented (in women) with implants (*augmentation mammaplasty*) to enhance the shape and size of the breast and/or with a breast lift, or mastopexy, a procedure that reduces the skin and literally lifts the breasts up. Implants and mastopexy are generally not covered by insurance companies. The scarring in women is frequently hidden in the crease underneath the breast. In men, however, the scarring is more apparent. The surgery becomes a trade-off for men; while it reduces the skin, there will likely be visible scars.

FACE/NECK/CHIN
Jowls, pouchy neck skin, and a flabby jawline are some residuals from significant weight loss and skin inelasticity. While many of these characteristics are age-related, weight loss can exacerbate the problem.

The Cosmetic Fix
The main facial procedure that addresses sagging facial skin, jowls, and loose neck skin is the face-lift, or *rhytidectomy*. The procedure removes excess skin, tightening muscles and redraping the skin of the face; it is generally not covered by insurance companies.

ARMS/LEGS
The arms of someone post-weight-loss are sometimes the most difficult body part to hide. The sagging skin can droop like bat wings, making it impossible for someone who has lost a lot of weight to wear tank tops or bathing suits without feeling self-conscious.

The Cosmetic Fix
The surgery used to treat this, a *brachioplasty*, or arm lift, involves an incision (and subsequent scar) from the underarm area all the way down the inside of the upper arm. Legs are treated similarly with a *thighplasty*, or thigh lift, but the scarring tends to be slightly less obvious. Arm and leg cosmetic procedures are generally not covered by insurance companies.

If you think cosmetic surgery will save you the trouble of going to the gym, think again, says Dr. Kleinman. All cosmetic procedures should be combined with muscle toning before and after the surgeries in order to maximize the effect. Of course, a reasonable recovery time comes with each procedure, but afterward, use your weights to keep on sculpting.

Cosmetic surgery is pricey, but if you figure out the cost of all the food you are no longer buying, and the fat clothes, you may be able to rationalize spending the money on yourself. According to Dr. Kleinman, a total body tightening can cost upwards of $20,000. Financing options through the plastic surgeon's office are becoming more available to help patients pay for the procedures.

CHOOSING A DOCTOR

Dr. Kleinman suggests that, in choosing a doctor to perform your plastic surgery, you consider the guidelines established by the American Society of Plastic Surgeons.

Doctors should:

- Have at least five years of surgical training and a minimum of two years of plastic surgery training.
- Be board-certified by the American Board of Plastic Surgery or the Royal College of Physicians and Surgeons of Canada.
- Be trained and experienced in all plastic surgery procedures, including breast, body, face, and reconstruction.
- Be peer-reviewed for safety and ethical standards prior to attaining the honor of active membership.
- Operate only in accredited facilities.

WHAT PLASTIC SURGERY DOESN'T FIX

Dr. Kleinman warns that realistic expectations are important when considering post-weight-loss plastic surgery. Don't expect:

- To suddenly look like a twenty-year-old model if you're forty-six.
- Liposuction to take fat off muscular body parts.
- Tummy tucks to create a six-pack abdomen. Internal fat cannot be removed.
- The skin to shrink completely.

"At some point, a person has to accept his or her own genetic makeup and know that he or she cannot be compared to anyone else," states Dr. Kleinman. "Someone who accepts his or her own potential and understands realistically what he or she can become is the ideal candidate for post-weight-loss plastic surgery."

Larina cautions that you should keep a realistic perspective on what plastic surgery does and doesn't fix. Many people feel understandably frustrated about loose, sagging skin after weight loss. They see plastic surgery as the last step to the perfect body and, therefore, to a perfect life. While plastic surgery may be your important step for entrance into The Thin Club and for your happiness with your physical appearance, it is not a cure-all; it will not fix everything.

Remember that "thin" does not equate to a perfect life. People still have many of the same difficulties once they are thin and free of sagging skin as they had when they were heavy. So they have the skin removed and maybe a couple other nips and tucks, and they expect everything will suddenly be great. Of course, this unrealistic expectation results in frustration and disappointment.

TIP

Figure out what the plastic surgery will and will not change. This exercise works best before you have the plastic surgery, but it can also be done afterward. List all the things you can think of that you are dissatisfied with or would like to improve upon. Brainstorm and dream a little to picture your life as you really want it to be. Once you have your list, circle all of the things that you can realistically change with plastic surgery. Then go through and put a star next to the things you can change with exercise. Everything that's left over is unlikely to be affected by exercise or surgery. Don't neglect these last things—come up with ways to improve them, too!

AVOIDING ADDICTION

You've seen all the recent media reports about addictions to plastic surgery. People return to plastic surgeons many times, or even dozens of times, for more and more procedures. "Beautiful people" make themselves look frightening by overdoing the plastic surgery. But plastic surgery can become addictive, because you get the initial high from the great change or improvement. Once you get used to it, the high wears off and you notice other "flaws," so you return again for more work. It is not a true addiction because your brain chemistry is not being altered by a substance, but people can become obsessed with plastic surgery and not know when to stop. You can lose your sound judgment and end up pursuing expensive procedures that are not only unnecessary but also risky for your mental and physical health, not to mention destructive to your appearance.

Larina cautions people who have lost a significant amount of weight that they can be at risk for plastic surgery "addiction." As you watch the pounds come off and your body transforms, you become used to the reinforcing cycle of observing appearance change based on your actions. Once you've lost the weight, you may substitute plastic surgery for dieting. This way, you continue to experience the feel-good process of physical transformation. You enjoyed the big "reveal" of the new you, and you want some more moments like that. Of course, this may come at a cost and you could sacrifice your hard-earned savings or go into debt, or put yourself at risk to keep up your makeover habit.

Remember that plastic surgery is a positive, viable option for some people who want to tie up loose ends or remove excess skin following dramatic weight loss. It is sometimes not necessary and even for those it helps, there is a limit to the amount of surgeries that are useful and beneficial. Bestselling motivation author Stephen Covey says to "begin with the end in mind." This is a good principle to apply to your plastic-surgery pursuits because it will show you when you are done and need to stop.

If you are not sure whether your interest in plastic surgery is out of control, get second and third opinions. An ethical plastic surgeon will let you know how much is too much and that you are entering the "proceed with caution" or "don't even think about anymore" zones. A psychologist can also help you determine whether you're developing an unhealthy obsession or if you're showing signs of body dysmorphic disorder, a condition that causes people to magnify perceived flaws that others often don't see.

TIP

Have you found a new way to do things to excess after you stopped eating in excess? Take an honest look at your exercise and plastic-surgery behaviors and plans. Think about whether you are taking something healthy, like exercise, to an extreme or you are finding yourself obsessed with it in a way that creates distress or disturbance in your life or for those close to you. Would someone else view your exercise or plastic-surgery preoccupation as excessive? If so, consider reevaluating how much you'll do these, and use the time and money you save to pursue some other healthy activity choices, like taking an art class, getting communications training or career coaching, or beginning a new hobby.

WHAT I DECIDED TO DO

I did visit a plastic surgeon. After looking me over he said, "You're in terrific shape," and he assured me, "It's an easy fix!"

Easy, he explained, involved chopping off my belly, restructuring my belly button, stretching my skin like a girdle across my pelvis, wearing post-operative drains, and a recovery that meant no kickboxing or rigorous exercise for weeks. I considered the options. Smooth, supple belly, or surgery? Um . . . no!

But I did finally decide to try something. Month after month of push-ups with a belly that drooped and dragged and knowing I had done about all that I could to lose the pouch was frustrating.

MESOTHERAPY: AN ALTERNATIVE TREATMENT

I found myself on a table in Dr. Shah's office experiencing needle after needle of amino acids being injected directly into those leftover fat cells—the same amino acids, like L-Carnitine, that I have been taking orally for years now. The treatment, which is still experimental here in the United States, is called mesotherapy and is said to help spot fat reduction for love handles, the abdomen, or other problematic areas.

According to Dr. Shah, many people end up with these areas after weight loss due to the anatomical distribution of the alpha and beta receptors in the subcutaneous tissue. Alpha receptors attract fat in an area as beta receptors eliminate the fat. The distribution of these receptors (particularly where the alpha receptors exist in a quantity that is much greater than that of the beta receptors) is what causes fat accumulation.

Males tend to have more alpha receptors and fewer beta receptors in the abdomen, therefore causing them to have bellies. Females typically have more alpha receptors in the thighs and buttocks regions. This treatment is said to help stimulate the beta receptors in a given area, causing them to eliminate fat even if the alpha receptor population is greater.

Dr. Shah says these injections should not be regarded as a new miracle drug for weight reduction and are only appropriate in the case of fat deposits that cannot be removed by diet or exercise.

The first treatment went well. I was examined thoroughly by Dr. Shah. He took my BMI, did bloodwork and an ECG, and checked all my vital signs carefully. After he gave me a clean bill of health, his assistant slathered my blown-out belly with numbing cream. Twenty minutes later, Dr. Shah injected the special cocktail of chemicals designed to kill off the bad cells. Yes, my diet had shrunk the cells, but this was going to eliminate them.

I went home that night in excruciating pain. My hanging belly was now swollen and varying shades of purple, blue, green, and yellow. "What was I thinking?" I wondered to myself. The pain and discoloration lasted a few days. One week later, though, I was amazed to look in the mirror and see a difference. My belly had changed shape! Dr. Shah measured me in his office. I was one inch smaller!

"More!" I demanded. He predicts that by the end of several treatments, my belly fat will shrink by four inches. And I didn't have to miss more than one day of kickboxing! So far, so good.

I'LL KEEP MY JIGGLE, THANKS

For those who don't elect to have surgery, keep the faith. You can certainly work on using exercise to tone as much as you can, and rest assured that you will look much better than you did pre-weight-loss. Bellies and hip skin can be cinched in with smoothies. When I was on *The Today Show,* a stylist recommended Spanx, a footless control-top garment that she called, "lipo in a package."

But the most important thing is to know that, whatever you have chosen to do about loose skin, you are a success story. Feel good, knowing that with or without help from a physician or from a control top, you are looking your best just by being thinner.

HOME FREE

How You Know
You're Thin for Life

ALL THAT WORK, BOTH PHYSICALLY AND MENTALLY—
how do you know you're really thinking like a thin person? How do you know when you have finally joined The Thin Club for life?

You know where you've been and where you've made it to, and you don't want to go back. Why would you? You've overcome many hurdles and accomplished so much that you deserve to stay and enjoy what you've created. But you can't help but wonder how long it will last and whether you'll continue to enjoy your membership for years to come.

ARE WE THERE YET?

As with most things in life, there's no guarantee that you'll be in The Thin Club forever, but there are some good predictors whether you'll stay a member. After reading this book, you now know the big ones, and we'll reveal a couple more in this chapter. First, take this quiz to test your Thin Club knowledge and ongoing membership potential. Answer each question with a yes or no:

1. I am pleased with myself for my journey downward and my ongoing commitment to being fit and healthy.
2. If eating had a deeper meaning for me, I've worked on those underlying issues.
3. I have conquered (or at least I'm dealing with) my fear of the fat coming back.
4. After losing the weight, I have set specific new goals for my weight and fitness.
5. I have or I'm making progress toward achieving a healthy body image.
6. I've adopted the attitudes toward food of those who've been successful at keeping the weight off.
7. I know how to handle emotional eating and have a list of many great activities to do instead of eating in response to certain emotions.
8. If I slip up and make a less healthy food choice, I don't berate myself. Instead, I simply make a plan to get back on track and implement it right away.
9. I have a strong support network of people who want me to stay in The Thin Club.
10. I've found ways to live in and enjoy the present, and I seize the opportunities each day brings.
11. I have a motivating exercise routine that involves both resistance training and cardiovascular exercise.
12. I believe my mind is becoming toned toward fitness along with my body.
13. I know that I have the right to dress tight and present myself as the attractive person I am.
14. I am able to graciously accept compliments and say "thank you" when someone tells me that I look great.
15. I have addressed relationship and intimacy problems that were around before I lost the weight or that came up following my weight loss.

16. I have figured out how to use or not use plastic
    surgery and exercise to complete my process.
17. I accept myself for who I am and how I look right now.
18. I am a proud card-carrying member of The Thin Club
    and I intend to stay a member!

How did you do? If you answered yes to most of the questions, then you're likely to remain a Thin Club member for life. With the last couple steps that we'll offer in this chapter, you can be assured that you'll have your membership, a fit body, and a toned mind for good.

Once you've mastered the last ideas we're about to discuss, you'll really be in great shape. Remember that ongoing membership does take some work and a *lot* of motivation and dedication, so don't get the idea that you can coast along now that things are going well. But as you know at this point, the rewards are worth the work. With each new day of your Thin Club membership, you'll prove even more that you've earned it and you belong!

If you answered no to many questions, then you may want to read this book again, pursue counseling or coaching, or take up a couple of other activities to ensure your membership. Thin is hard to achieve but harder to stay, so it's crucial that you give yourself the best chance to enjoy this new body and life that you have created for yourself.

THE LAST TEN POUNDS

"So how much weight do you still want to lose?" The doctor I was interviewing for a magazine article surveyed me critically. I had shown her my "before" photos proudly.

"Well, I could lose another ten, I suppose," I told her. "Or maybe I won't. Whatever I do, I know I won't gain. That's what matters most to me."

She stared, and wrinkled her brow. Was that the wrong answer? Am I there yet? Not in her book, perhaps, but in mine I am.

That darn scale is a fickle beast. No sooner do I think that I know it all than it goes up a pound. No sooner do I reaffirm that I can do it than I manage to bring it down again. It's that last ten pounds—the ones that will put me into a comfortable size 6—that seem to elude me. It can't just be a plateau because I've been the same weight—give or take a pound or two of occasional water gain and loss—for a couple of years now. I just don't seem to be getting any closer to losing them.

Alarmed, I went back to Rosie. She told me not to sweat it—that the only real way to lose that final ten is to embrace lettuce like a bunny and never, ever give myself even the occasional indulgent bite of something sweet, starchy, or remotely carb-laden, even if it is high in fiber. "At this point, it's a matter of choices," she explained. "You can choose to lose that final ten, but you will have to be disciplined—more disciplined than you've been—forever, of course. Or you can know that your body has found its set point. It's healthy and you're thin."

Yeah, *but* . . . what about that coworker who was describing his ultra-thin wife. "She has a model's size two figure," he crowed. "She is the type of woman whom the designers make clothing for." I dared to argue. Size 2 hardly appears to be the norm—in fact, even a "large" size 8 seems tiny when you're shopping for clothes in a world that seems to be getting larger all the time. And designers are not blind. They want to be where the volume is because volume translates into money.

And as I caught myself defending my "large" size 8, I contemplated slapping the man who was somehow making me feel fat. Have I learned nothing from all my experiences? Have I learned nothing from writing this book? Was there any other way of letting the world know—letting myself know—that I am a thin person? But I knew the culprit wasn't the man with the stick-thin wife. It was me, me, me! I wasn't "there" yet!

So I decided to do something that many women might find horrifying: pose for a nude photo.

I've taken so many photographs over the course of my lifetime. It sounds simple, staring at the camera under bright lights at a photographer that I've known for years—my fishing buddy, in fact. I smiled without a care as he snapped my photograph. I've had many pictures taken of me before. He did my last book photos. But as I dared to bare it all for a nude photo shoot that photographer Robert Buchanan was taking for his own book—an exhibit of women over forty, in their semi-nude splendor—I realized just how far I'd really come.

I had dressed carefully that day—don't ask me why, since I wasn't going to be wearing anything but my shoes, some carefully positioned fabric, and those ever-present stretch marks. I kept in mind that high heels always make legs look slimmer. As I walked into the lights, draped in a Roberto Cavalli silk print fabric, I wondered if I would have the nerve to let it go. Bob stood behind the camera, waiting patiently. And then I realized: I wanted to let go. Yeah, I had lumps and feminine bumps, and of course I didn't look like a size 2 model, but I was proud of what I'd become. I knew where I'd been, I knew I looked good, but more important, I was positive about where I was going. And it was all good. This body was a gift from God and my parents. It is my legacy to care for and it is insurance for my children. My arms may not be pencil-like scrawny, but they give great hugs. And those stretch marks—each one was earned. And look at the three great kids that belly, now slightly droopy, had produced. I may not be "the best," but I knew without a doubt that I was the best that I can be—the best I'd ever been—and I was damn proud of it.

So I dropped the drape and I posed and I smiled. And amazingly, it didn't feel one bit weird. In fact, it felt fabulous. I was thin. I was beautiful. I was happy with what I'd become. And I was never going back.

THE ART OF ACCEPTANCE

The day I accidentally turned on a red light and the hunky thirty-something police officer approached to give me a ticket, I turned on my charm, apologized profusely, and used all the "girly" skills I once thought were repugnant. He looked at the very flustered lady, and he winked.

"I'll let you off with a warning this time," he said sternly. I played my role with all the ingénue power I could muster. "Oh, thank you *so* much, Officer," my cleavage heaving in relief (not too faked—it was a $250 ticket!) at the reprieve. He nodded and I gave him a grateful smile. Wow, I love flirting; where has it been all these years? And where have *I* been all these years? Hiding behind layers of unattractive fat, that's where. And whether I whip out the fat pictures or not, these last few years have been my "coming out" party. I know it—and that's all that matters.

I feel much the same way as Sally Field did when she delivered her famous acceptance speech at the Oscars, "You like me—you really, really like me!" Only I'm not looking for love and approval from anyone else—not my friends, family, boyfriend, parents, not even from the scale. I can finally look in the mirror (or at my photos) and state definitively, "I like me. I *really, really* like me!"

Even if you're not quite to the point of liking where you are, that's OK. What's important is that you accept yourself and work on liking yourself a little bit more each day. Focus on all the incredible work you've done to help you: You've defied the odds and made it into The Thin Club, and that is something to feel good about! One of the most important variables in the process of weight loss is *acceptance,* even if you're not quite ready to love the extra pounds, skin, and bulges. Accepting yourself *regardless of eating and weight problems* is very important and very difficult to do.

One of the most important times to call on your acceptance skills is when you've done something that threatens your Thin Club membership. It is natural to judge ourselves when we make an unhealthy food choice. You might think, "I am so weak—how did I cave in and eat that whole pizza?" or "I have no control or willpower. I am powerless against a bag of cookies; how pathetic!" Thoughts like these are a normal response; however, these types of thoughts can sabotage your membership.

The best test of your self-acceptance is when you actually make a "mistake." You may not love yourself when you're feeling bloated after partaking of too many New Year's Eve cocktails, but it is vital that you don't negatively judge yourself. Everyone makes good choices and bad choices from time to time. If you make mostly good, healthy choices, then don't worry—your Thin Club membership won't be threatened.

Work to accept yourself in all aspects of your life, not just your weight loss. And when you mess up, take that as an opportunity to learn a lesson. Larina likes to say that because problem and opportunity are two sides of the same coin, you have a choice: If you get a problem, you can flip it over and see the opportunity.

For example, if you overeat at one meal, you can take that as an opportunity to prove to yourself that you can get right back on track. If you miss a day at the gym, you can do some push-ups at home or go to a class the next day and show yourself that you're serious about managing your weight and being healthy. The vehicle that helps you turn problems into opportunities is acceptance. Without it, you'll be stuck in place or you may even start slipping backward.

And to me, that's what being in The Thin Club is all about: acceptance. I'm not perfect, not by a long shot. But I am most certainly thin. Maybe not as thin as I could be, but certainly thin enough to be healthy and not be considered by most of the world as fat. And for those who do think I'm large—well, let them think what they want. There will always be critics. There will be those who say I'm too fat, too thin, too sexy, too outspoken. But they don't matter. I feel great knowing that I am caring for myself to the best of my ability. I am keeping my body fueled, tuned, fit, and satisfied. I have learned not to listen to others, but to heed my own inner voice.

Turn down the volume of the critical inner voice and turn up the volume of the inspirational inner voice. You can be your own best champion. You can go out and do all the things you're meant to do. You can live your dreams. You can commit to remain in The Thin Club for life. You can do it all—you know you can because you've already achieved an amazing accomplishment. You've toned your mind and body.

To me, that is what being thin is all about. It is not a number. It is not a size. It is an overall commitment to taking care of your body through diet and exercise. It's embracing the notion of being thin. It's about knowing that food is neither friend nor foe, but fuel. If you use it to maximize your energy, you will gain not weight but the ability to effect physical and mental achievements that you never dreamed possible.

The Thin Club is about taking away the power of food to victimize and giving it the power to energize. Most important, realize that you are the only person who has the ability to victimize yourself. Once you absorb that message, food is powerless, and the people or situations that drove you to eat are ineffective. Once you absorb that message, you become a card-carrying member of The Thin Club.

Visit our website, www.thethinclub.com, to join this select club and share *your* victories, because becoming thin—while sometimes a work in progress—is always, and we do mean *always,* a victory. Congratulations!

RESOURCES

The Thin Club Site

www.thethinclub.com
Get membership tips, tell us your stories, and join the club.

Websites with Free Resources

www.strengthweightloss.com
Larina's company site offers dozens of free articles, tools, and resources. Get a free eight-week e-course revealing the STRENGTH formula when you enroll in the STRENGTH *Insider Newsletter.*

http://weightloss.about.com/
A site with many great resources and links about different diets and weight loss.

www.weightlosssurgeryinfo.com/
Explore different options related to weight-loss surgery.

http://obesityhelp.com
This site has many great resources pre- and post-weight-loss surgery.

www.pale-reflections.com/
A site for eating-disorder support, referrals, and information on eating problems.

www.betterwaypress.com/dietsurvivors/
This site has many great articles on the nondieting
approach to weight loss.

www.something-fishy.org/
This is a website for help with eating disorders, including
compulsive overeating.

www.bodypositive.com/
Resources for boosting your body image at any weight.

www.about-face.org/
This is an organization that helps build self-esteem for
women and girls of all ages.

Further Reading

Books on Eating

Albers, S. 2003. *Eating Mindfully: How to End Mindless Eating
and Enjoy a Balanced Relationship with Food.* Oakland,
Calif.: New Harbinger Publications.

Fairburn, C. 1995. *Overcoming Binge Eating.* New York:
Guilford Press.

Rippe, J. M., and Weight Watchers. 2004. *WeightWatchers®
Weight Loss That Lasts: Break Through the 10 Big Diet
Myths.* New York: John Wiley & Sons.

Somer, E. 1999. *Food & Mood: The Complete Guide to Eating
Well and Feeling Your Best.* 2nd ed. New York: Owl Books.

Tribole, E., and E. Resch. 2003. *Intuitive Eating: A
Revolutionary Program That Works.* New York: St. Martin's
Press.

Weil, A. 2001. *Eating Well for Optimal Health.* New York:
HarperCollins.

Books on Weight-Loss Surgery

Janeway, J. M., and K. J. Sparks. 2005. *The Real Skinny on Weight Loss Surgery: An Indispensable Guide to What You Can Really Expect!* Onondaga, Mich.: Little Victoria Press.

Leach, S. M. 2004. *Before and After: Living and Eating Well After Weight Loss Surgery.* New York: HarperCollins.

Books on Body Image and Self-Esteem

Cash, T. F. 1997. *The Body Image Workbook: An 8-Step Program for Learning to Like Your Looks.* Oakland, Calif.: New Harbinger Publications.

Cooke-Kearney, A. 2004. *Change Your Mind, Change Your Body—Feeling Good About Your Body and Self After 40.* New York: Atria Books.

Freedman, R. 2002. *Bodylove—Learning to Like Our Looks and Ourselves.* Carlsbad, Calif.: Gurze Books.

Johnson, C. 2002. *Self-Esteem Comes in All Sizes—How to Be Happy and Healthy at Your Natural Weight.* Carlsbad, Calif.: Gurze Books.

Sell, C. 2003. *Yoga from the Inside Out: Making Peace with Your Body Through Yoga.* Prescott, Ariz.: Hohm Press.

Wilhelm, S. 2006. *Feeling Good about the Way You Look: A Program for Overcoming Body Image Problems.* New York: Guilford Press.

Cookbooks

Daelemans, K. 2002. *Cooking Thin with Chef Kathleen: 200 Easy Recipes for Healthy Weight Loss.* New York: Houghton Mifflin.

Levine, P., and M. Bontmpo-Saray. 2004. *Eating Well After Weight Loss Surgery: Over 140 Delicious Low-Fat,*

High-Protein Recipes to Enjoy in the Weeks, Months and Years After Surgery. New York: Marlowe & Company.

Weight Watchers International Inc. Staff. 2006. *Weight Watchers New Complete Cookbook.* New York: John Wiley & Sons.

Find a Therapist

http://locator.apahelpcenter.org/
   The American Psychological Association's directory of psychologists.

www.pale-reflections.com/treatment_finder.asp
   A good guide for finding therapists.

www.aabt.org
   The Association for the Advancement of Behavioral Therapy provides links for finding cognitive-behavioral therapists.

NOTES

INTRODUCTION
Joining the Thin Club

Realistic Weight-Loss Goals

11   In clinical studies, the goal for weight loss at the end of treatment is typically around 10 percent of your initial body weight.

Quality-of-Life Improvement

13   *Studies typically show an improved quality of life.* . . . Choban, P. S., J. Onyejekwe, J. C. Burge, and L. Flancbaum. 1999. A health status assessment of the impact of weight loss following Roux-en-Y gastric bypass for clinically severe obesity. *Journal of the American College of Surgeons, 188:* 491–497.

Weight Regain

5   . . . *95 percent of people who lose large amounts of weight* . . . Institute of Medicine (IOM). 1995. *Weighing the Options: Criteria for Evaluating Weight-Management Programs.* Washington, D.C.: National Academy Press. Also, Cooper and Fairburn (as cited in Wadden & Stunkard, below) are two eminent scholars in weight loss and body image who advocate ongoing maintenance (addressing body image, long-term goals, and regular exercise and healthy eating) for long-term weight loss. Wadden T. A., and A. J. Stunkard (Eds.). 2004.

Handbook of Obesity Treatment. New York: Guilford Press.

15   . . . *unrealistic expectations for how much weight* . . . Foster, G. D., T. A. Wadden, R. A. Vogt, and G. Brewer. 1997. What is a reasonable weight loss?: Patients' expectations and evaluation of obesity treatment outcomes. *Journal of Consulting and Clinical Psychology, 65:* 79–85.

ONE

Against All Odds
How I Made the Journey Downscale

37   Judy's weight-loss plan was supervised by Rosie Schulman, RN. Learn more about her at www.tipping thescalesforyou.com.

TWO

Fear of the Fat Coming Back

See Introduction notes for studies referencing weight regain.

52   *In an interesting study, researchers led men* . . . Snyder, M., E. D. Tank, and E. Berscheid. 1977. Social perception and interpersonal behaviour: On the self-fulfilling nature of social stereotypes. *Journal of Personality and Social Psychology, 35:* 656–666.

57   For studies on processing fears, see the seminal article: Foa, E. B., and M. J. Kozak. 1986. Emotional processing of fear: Exposure to corrective information. *Psychological Bulletin, 99*(1): 20–35.

Cognitive therapy concepts to address the distortions in thinking when people are anxious can be found in books such as: Beck, A. T. 1976. *Cognitive Therapy and*

the Emotional Disorders. New York: Penguin; Burns, D.
D. 1980. *Feeling Good: The New Mood Therapy*. New
York: Quill.

THREE

Your Relationship with Food
Addressing the Hidden Meanings

68 *When people are emotionally, physically, or sexually* . . .
Studies have shown a link between childhood
abuse and adult obesity: Felitti, V. J., R. F. Anda,
D. Nordenberg, D. F. Williamson, A. M. Spitz,
V. Edwards, M. P. Koss, and J. S. Marks. 1998.
Relationship of childhood abuse and household
dysfunction to many of the leading causes of death
in adults: The Adverse Childhood Experiences (ACE)
Study. *American Journal of Preventative Medicine*,
14: 245–258.

71 Research by Dr. Edna Foa and colleagues has shown
that effective treatments for trauma involve
confronting and experiencing memories of the
traumatic event: Rothbaum, B. O., and E. B. Foa. 1993.
Subtypes of posttraumatic stress disorder and duration
of symptoms. In: J. R. T. Davidson and E. B. Foa (Eds.),
Posttraumatic Stress Disorder: DSM-IV and Beyond (pp.
23–35). Washington, D.C.: American Psychiatric Press;
Foa, E. B., and B. O. Rothbaum. 1998. *Treating the
Trauma of Rape: Cognitive-Behavioral Therapy for PTSD*.
New York: Guilford Press.

74 For therapy referrals to address trauma or anxiety, see
Association for the Advancement of Behavioral
Therapy (provides links for finding cognitive-
behavioral therapists; www.aabt.org).

74   Find links to resources related to traumatic stress on page from the International Society for Traumatic Stress Studies, http://istss.org/resources/traumatic_stress.htm.

75   Several studies have shown that prolonged-exposure therapy (a type of cognitive-behavioral therapy) is highly effective in reducing symptoms of PTSD; see Foa, E. B., and E. A. Meadows. 1997. Psychosocial treatments for post-traumatic stress disorder: A critical review. In: J. Spence, J. M. Darley, and D. J. Foss (Eds.), *Annual Review of Psychology, 28* (pp. 449–480). Palo Alto, Calif.: Annual Reviews.

FOUR

When the Goal Is Gone
Creating New Goals to Keep You Inspired

81   *Top researchers in the treatment of obesity* . . . Research at Oxford University and other research and treatment centers has shown the importance of ongoing treatment in maintaining weight loss over the long term: Cooper, Z., C. G. Fairburn, and D. M. Hawker. 2003. *Cognitive-Behavioral Treatment of Obesity: A Clinician's Guide.* New York: Guilford Press.

83   *Once you select some goals* . . . It is unknown who came up with the concept of SMART goals, but they have been effectively used in a variety of contexts, from sports psychology to career advancement to weight loss.

FIVE

Cut the Criticism
Building a Better Body Image

91   *Your body image is your relationship with your body.*
      Information in the two paragraphs following this
      sentence is adapted from: Cash, T. 1995. *What Do You
      See When You Look in the Mirror? Helping Yourself to a
      Positive Body Image.* New York: Bantam Books.

95   *In a study, those who were overweight or obese as teens . . .*
      Obesity earlier in life is associated with a negative body
      image after weight loss: Adami, G. F., P. Gandolfo,
      B. Bauer, and N. Scopinaro. 1995. Binge eating in
      massively obese patients undergoing bariatric surgery.
      International Journal of Eating Disorders, 17: 45–50.

95   Studies have shown that body image typically improves
      with small amounts of weight loss, but that larger
      amounts of weight loss are not associated with greater
      improvements in body image. There is no direct
      relationship between body image and weight or weight
      loss: Brown, T. A., T. F. Cash, and P. J. Mikulka. 1990.
      Attitudinal body image assessment: Factor analysis of
      the Body-Self Relations Questionnaire. *Journal of
      Personality Assessment, 55:* 135–144.

96   *. . . changing your thinking and behavior can lead . . .*
      Rosen, J. C., P. Orosan, and J. Reiter. 1995. Cognitive
      behavior therapy for negative body image in obese
      women. *Behavior Therapy, 26:* 25–42.

97   *. . . a negative body image can persist even after weight
      has come off.* Cash, T. F., B. Counts, and C. E. Huffine.
      1990. Current and vestigial effects of overweight among
      women: Fear of fat, attitudinal body image, and eating
      behaviors. *Journal of Psychopathology and Behavioral
      Assessment, 12:* 157–167.

SIX

Risky Times
Dealing with Backslide Temptations

110   *"When you get a flat tire, you fix it or replace the tire and keep on going," he says.* Steve Olschwanger is certified as a Master Trainer in Physical Fitness and Nutrition, and he works with a method that combines a unique style of nutritional and physical fitness information with motivation.

111   *Findings from a research study at the Rush University Medical Center in Chicago showed that . . .* This study was conducted with 2,000 women at Rush University Medical Center.

112   *If you haven't learned how to break the association . . .* Find resources for ending emotional eating at www.Ending EmotionalEating.com.

114   *Do the opposite and confront what . . .* This is a common theory in cognitive-behavioral therapy for treating depression, anxiety, and other psychological problems, put forth by researchers such as Dr. Marsha Linehan: Linehan, M. M. 1993. *Skills Training Manual for Treating Borderline Personality Disorder.* New York: Guilford Press.

SEVEN

Staying Fit
Developing Exercise Routines You Can Stick With

123   *Research by the National Institutes of Health and the National Heart, Lung and Blood Institute indicates that . . .* National Institutes of Health and National Heart, Lung and Blood Institute. 1998. *Obesity Education Initiative:*

Clinical Guidelines on the Identification, Evaluation, and Treatment of Overweight and Obesity in Adults. Bethesda, Md.: U.S. Department of Health and Human Services.

123 *Research shows that those who stick to an exercise regimen . . .* Blair and Leemaker found that when people who kept weight off and people who were "normal" weight both exercise regularly, regular physical activity is an important factor for both groups. Cited in: Wadden, T. A., and A. J. Stunkard (Eds.). 2004. *Handbook of Obesity Treatment.* New York: Guilford Press.

124 *. . . results of a three-year study of men showed that . . .* Pavlou, K. N., S. Krey, and W. P. Steffee. 1989. Exercise as an adjunct to weight loss and maintenance in moderately obese subjects. *America Journal of Clinical Nutrition, 49*(5 suppl): 1115–1123.

127 *Research shows that resistance exercise may . . .* Andersen, R. E., and J. M. Jakicic. 2003. Physical activity and weight management: Building the case for exercise. *The Physician and Sports Medicine Online, 31*(9).

128 *One research team found that formerly obese women . . .* Schoeller D. A., K. Shay, and R. F. Kushner. 1997. How much physical activity is needed to minimize weight gain in previously obese women? *America Journal of Clinical Nutrition, 66*(3): 551–556.

138 *Cynthia Sass, a dietitian and the coauthor . . .* Sass, C., and D. Maher. 1994. *Your Diet Is Driving Me Crazy: When Food Conflicts Get in the Way of Your Love Life.* New York: Marlowe & Company.

EIGHT

Friends and Foes
Developing a Positive Support Network

150   *Here's a multiple-choice quiz* . . . This quiz was created by
         Larina Kase for this book.

157   *A great way to meet new friends* . . . We recommend that
         readers search on the Internet for clubs and activities
         in their local areas. For example, someone in San Diego
         who's interested in meeting active people can search
         for "runner's clubs San Diego" or "mountain biking
         groups San Diego."

169   *Many people find support groups run by organizations* . . .
         You can learn more about these on Weight Watchers'
         site, www.weightwatchers.com. You can find many
         great food ideas and recipes and success stories on
         their website as well.

170   *Individual therapy is a powerful vehicle* . . . You can get
         more information or find a therapist on sites such as
         those for the Anxiety Disorders Association of America
         (www.adaa.org) or the Association for the
         Advancement of Behavioral Therapy (www.aabt.org).

173   *Many coaches possess certifications* . . . You can also
         learn more about coaching at the ICF website, www.
         coachfederation.org.

ELEVEN

Shopping
Dressing the New You

198   *Larina cites a study that shows that 73 percent* . . . Cash,
         T. F., B. Counts, and C. E. Huffine. 1990. Current and
         vestigial effects of overweight among women: Fear of
         fat, attitudinal body image, and eating behaviors.

Journal of Psychopathology and Behavioral Assessment,
12: 157–167.

202   *"Don't grab everything in sight," urges stylist James Aguiar.*
James Aguiar is a celebrity stylist and professional
shopper who has appeared on numerous television
shows. He helps people improve their fashion choices.

FOURTEEN

The Skinny on Sex

235   *According to Cynthia Sass . . .* Sass, C., and D. Maher.
1994. *Your Diet Is Driving Me Crazy: When Food Conflicts*
Get in the Way of Your Love Life. New York: Marlowe &
Company.

236   *But according to Christine Ren, a surgeon . . .* Information
gathered from a personal interview, January 2006.

238   *According to Dr. Bartlik . . .* Information gathered from a
personal interview, January 2006.

241   *If you spot verbally abusive or controlling behaviors . . .*
For more information on the free National Domestic
Violence Hotline, see www.ndvh.org.

FIFTEEN

Loose Ends
Plastic Surgery

246   *Andrew Kleinman, a board-certified plastic surgeon . . .*
Information gathered from a personal interview,
December 2005.

253   *Bestselling motivation author Stephen Covey says to . . .*
Covey, S. 2004. *The 7 Habits of Highly Effective People.*
New York: Simon and Schuster.

ACKNOWLEDGMENTS

The teamwork that goes into writing a book is comparable to the team you learn to rely upon when finally committing to losing weight. Coaches, trainers, nutrition experts, friends, and families are all part of the process. And then, one day— you're there!

I thank God for sending me the myriad "messengers" to help me in my journey for health and fulfillment. Specifically, thanks to my coauthor, Larina Kase, for her impeccable attention to detail and for her personal advice that I've come to rely on, and to the minions at Random House and my team at The WAG who all contributed in some aspect to the production of this book. On the personal front, Jason, Eric, and Casey—you are sweeter than any dessert I've ever sampled and zero calories. Thank you to my mother and father who have always believed in me. Rosie Schulman, Nancy Adler, and Liz Holden were just a few of the friends who helped me get to a size 8. And one more big thanks to all my online muses—you know who you are!

Larina and I both want to thank our editor, Julia Pastore, and our agent, Faith Hamlin, who worked together and in separate ways to see to it that this book came to market.

—Judith Lederman

I would like to thank first and foremost, Judy Lederman for her captivating writing style, which made completing our book so much fun, and her openness about her own experiences, which I know will greatly help people. I also want to acknowledge the dedicated researchers in the field of obesity and binge eating including Albert J. Stunkard, Christopher Fairburn, and the others who've contributed so much to the field.

Finally I'd like to acknowledge my family for instilling a healthy lifestyle in me—my mom, who has taught me about healthy eating ever since she made her own hand-pureed baby food for me; my sister who regularly makes it to the gym despite a crazy schedule; my dad who's always up and about and is great with portion control; my incredibly active grandmother, Moraima; and my marathon-running husband, John.

To my clients, who know that getting and staying in The Thin Club is not easy, but that it is fun and definitely worth it!

—Larina Kase

INDEX

ABOUT THE AUTHORS

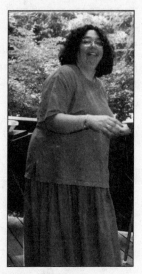

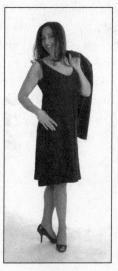

BEFORE   AFTER

Judith Lederman, mom of three, journalist, editor, entre-
preneur, and newly thin person, is the paradigm for second
chances and reinvention. As in her last book, *The Ups & Downs
of Raising a Bipolar Child: A Survival Guide for Parents* (Simon &
Schuster, 2003), Lederman uses frank anecdotes and witty wisdom to reach out to others who, like her, may need guidance,
reassurance, and support in coping with the psychological aftermath of weight loss. Judith is president of JSL Publicity &
Marketing, a Scarsdale-based public relations company. For more
information on Judith Lederman and *Joining the Thin Club,*
visit www.thethinclub.com.

Larina Kase, Psy.D., M.B.A. is a psychologist and the president of STRENGTH Weight Loss & Wellness. She specializes in helping women end emotional eating, achieve weight loss that lasts, balance work and life, and manage stress and anxiety. A regular in media such as *SELF* and *Marie Claire,* Dr. Kase enjoys sharing her ideas, and she provides wellness and stress management workshops to universities, organizations, and Fortune 500 companies. Visit her on the web at www.strengthweightloss.com or www.pascoaching.com.